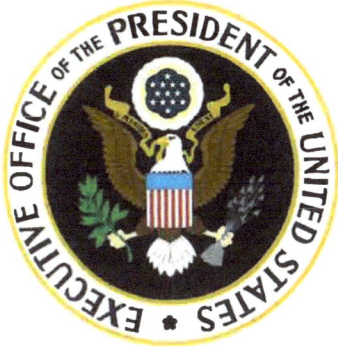

# PLAYBOOK FOR

# EARLY RESPONSE TO HIGH-CONSEQUENCE EMERGING INFECTIOUS DISEASE THREATS AND BIOLOGICAL INCIDENTS

## TABLE OF CONTENTS

## CHAPTER I – EXECUTIVE SUMMARY

I.      PLAYBOOK PURPOSE.................................................................................PAGE 04

II.     POLICY COORDINATION AND EXERCISING THE PLAYBOOK.............................PAGE 04

III.     RISK ASSESSMENT DASHBOARD................................................................PAGE 05

       A. INTERNATIONAL.................................................................................PAGE 06

       B. DOMESTIC........................................................................................PAGE 07

IV.     SAMPLE PATHOGENS INVOLVED..............................................................PAGE 08

V.      OTHER KEY CONSIDERATIONS.................................................................PAGE 11

## CHAPTER II – PLAYBOOK: DECISION-MAKING RUBRICS

I.      INTERNATIONAL....................................................................................PAGE 14

II.     DOMESTIC...........................................................................................PAGE 31

## CHAPTER III – APPENDIX MATERIAL

I.     DECLARATION AND MITIGATION OPTIONS...................................................PAGE 42

II.    KEY DEPARTMENTS AND AGENCIES..........................................................PAGE 46

       A. INTERNATIONAL.................................................................................PAGE 46

       B. DOMESTIC........................................................................................PAGE 52

III.   SAMPLE EXERCISES...............................................................................PAGE 62

IV.   COMMUNICATIONS................................................................................PAGE 67

V.    CONCEPT OF OPERATIONS FOR DOMESTIC RESPONSE.................................PAGE 68

# CHAPTER I – EXECUTIVE SUMMARY

## I.    Purpose of the Playbook

The goal of the Playbook For High-Consequence Emerging Infectious Disease Threats and Biological Incidents (Playbook) is to assist U.S. Government experts and leaders in coordinating a complex U.S. Government response to a high-consequence emerging disease threat anywhere in the world with the potential to cause an epidemic, pandemic, or other significant public health event, by providing a decision-making tool that identifies: (1) questions to ask; (2) agency counterparts to consult for answers to each; and (3) key decisions which may require deliberation through the Presidential Policy Directive (PPD)-1 process or its successor National Security Council process.  The Playbook also includes sample documents that can be used for interagency meetings that need to be called at each stage. While each emerging infectious disease threat will present itself in a unique way, a consistent, capabilities-based approach to addressing these threats will allow for faster decisions with more targeted expert subject matter input from Federal departments and agencies.

This Playbook is also intended to complement the Biological Incident Annex (BIA) of the Federal Interagency Operational Plans as well as the Department of Health and Human Services (HHS) Pandemic Influenza Crisis Action Plan (PANCAP).

This Playbook has two sections to assist with decision-making: (1) an international response rubric for emerging disease threats that start or are circulating in another country but not yet confirmed within United States territorial borders; and (2) a domestic response rubric drawn from the BIA and PANCAP that addresses emerging disease threats within our nation's borders.  Specific triggers for response actions and operational phases for both domestic and international emerging infectious disease threat incidents are outlined.  Each section of this Playbook includes specific questions that should be asked and decisions that should be made at multiple levels within the PPD-1 process or its successor National Security Council process.

## II.    Exercising the Playbook

Per PPD-1, the National Security Council (NSC) and its subordinate policy committees [including the Principals Committee (PC), the Deputies Committee (DC), and the Interagency Policy Committees (IPC)] will serve as the principal forum for consideration of national security policy issues, including emerging infectious disease-related national security threats. Departments and agencies should be regularly convened to review emerging infectious disease threats, as appropriate; highlight any situations that require closer watch, risk assessment, or experimental medical countermeasures (MCM); coordinate outreach and communications with key international stakeholders; inventory department and agency capabilities that can be deployed in various response situations; review infectious disease response planning, including communications on international and domestic response coordination; and regularly schedule exercises to improve interoperability and real-time decision making.  At a minimum, such meetings should consist of representatives from HHS (including the Centers for

Disease Control and Prevention (CDC), the National Institutes of Health (NIH), the Assistant Secretary for Preparedness and Response (ASPR), the Office of Global Affairs (OGA) and others), Department of Labor (DOL)/Occupational Safety and Health Administration (OSHA), Department of Defense (DOD), Department of Transportation (DOT), United States Agency for International Development (USAID), Department of State (DOS), Department of Homeland Security (DHS), United States Department of Agriculture (USDA), Environmental Protection Agency (EPA), and members of the Intelligence Community. Regular communications and joint meetings with the Domestic Resilience Group IPC (DRG) or its successor process and its member agencies should be established whenever a high-consequence emerging infectious disease threat has the potential to impact the United States.

In the event an infectious disease threat emerges or evolves rapidly or requires immediate decision-making, the Biological Incident Notification and Assessment (BINA) protocol will be used to convene all relevant departments and agencies.

## III.   Risk Assessment Dashboard

A key recommendation from the World Health Organization (WHO) is the need to assess the risk of an infectious disease threat before it becomes a Public Health Emergency of International Concern (PHEIC). Based on WHO risk assessment guidance, Table 1 and Table 2 provide dashboards intended to serve as guidance for discussion of how best to assess the risk of an evolving infectious disease threat along four critical dimensions: (1) epidemiology; (2) humanitarian/development/public health impact; (3) security/political stability; and (4) transmission/outbreak/potential for public concern in the United States.

There are several other epidemiologic risk assessment tools that exist for specific disease categories and that have clear criteria for assessing the level of threat. The following dashboards are not intended to supplant these tools, but are intended to overlay other security and humanitarian concerns to achieve a broader picture of the threat. Additionally, a dashboard is not intended to serve or replace a comprehensive risk assessment, but rather serve as a quick snapshot to inform policy makers' strategic decision making processes.

*The following tables govern United States decision-making in the event of an emerging infectious disease threat.*

Table 1: International Incident: Operational Phases & International Response Rubric

| Epidemiologic Rating→ | 1a. Normal Ops | 1b. Elevated Threat | 1c. Credible Threat | 2a. Public Health Emergency of International Concern / PHEIC | 2b. Worsening public health emergency indicators/ PHEIC | 2c. Improving public health emergency / PHEIC |
|---|---|---|---|---|---|---|
| Key Epidemiologic Rating | | | | | | |
| *Other Critical Dimensions* ↓ | | | | | | |
| Humanitarian/development/public health impact | | | | | | |
| Security/political indicators | | | | | | |
| Transmission/outbreak/potential for public concern in the US | | | | | | |
| **Overall Assessment** | | | | | | |

## Table 2: Domestic Incident: Phases, Stages, Triggering Events and Indicators for Response

| Phase | Phase I Primarily Pre-Incident | | | Phase 2 Begins Upon Notification When/After an Incident Occurs | | |
|---|---|---|---|---|---|---|
| **Phase** | 1a | 1b | 1c | 2a | 2b | 2c |
| **Rating** | **Normal Operations** | **Elevated Threat** | **Credible Threat** | Initial Response: Activation, Situational Assessment, and Movement | Employment of Resources and Stabilization | Intermediate Operations |
| **Triggering Events** | • No specific threat | • Identification of a human case of a high-consequence emerging infectious disease anywhere | • Confirmation of multiple human cases of a PPP anywhere<br><br>**AND/OR**<br><br>• Determination of a Significant Potential for a Public Health Emergency | • Demonstration of efficient and sustained human-to-human transmission of a novel virus anywhere<br><br>**AND/OR**<br><br>• Declaration of a Public Health Emergency | • Increasing number of cases in U.S. or healthcare system burden that exceed State resource<br><br>**AND/OR**<br><br>• State/local request for assistance | • Cases continue to climb with long term service disruption and critical infrastructure impacts<br><br>**AND/OR**<br><br>• Presidential Stafford Act declaration<br><br>**AND/OR**<br><br>• State/local request for assistance |
| **Key Epidemiologic Indicators** | | • Identification of a human case of a pathogen of pandemic potential | • Confirmation of multiple human cases | • Demonstration of efficient and sustained human to human transmission | | |
| **Humanitarian/ public health Impact Indicators** | | | | | | |
| **Security/Political Stability Indicators** | | | | | | |
| **Overall Risk Assessment** | | | | | | |

## IV.    Pathogens of Pandemic Potential Involved in Incident(s)

A newly emerging infectious disease pathogen may represent a high-consequence threat to human health, which at first may be unknown.  For instance, influenza poses a constant threat for emergence into an epidemic or pandemic.  Other pathogens have also recently emerged with little or no warning, such as Severe Acute Respiratory Syndrome (SARS), which was first reported in February 2003 and quickly spread to more than 20 countries before it was contained.  Determining the primary mode of transmission is critical during the early stages of an emerging infectious disease threat response.  However, this information may not be readily available.  Initial estimates are likely to be based on limited and incomplete information and will be continually reassessed based on new information.

Key questions about a pathogen that may affect the size, scale, and design of the response include:

1.  How is the pathogen transmitted? Can it be transmitted human-to-human, insects, or other animals and how can transmission be prevented or interrupted?

    Sources of information: HHS (ASPR, CDC, NIH), USDA

2.  What is the disease impact now and what do we know about its potential impact in the future?

    - Estimates on transmissibility and clinical severity

    - Forecasts and modeling

    Sources of information: HHS (ASPR, CDC, NIH)

3.  Can the disease be treated successfully?

    - Are there approved pharmaceutical interventions or experimental MCM in development?
    - Is the pathophysiology of the disease understood and can the disease be successfully treated using other forms of care?

    Sources of information: HHS (ASPR, CDC)

4.  Are there tools to mitigate the spread or disinfect contaminated surfaces?

    Sources of information: HHS (CDC, NIH), EPA, USDA

Pathogens that would cause heightened concern include, but are not limited to, novel (non-seasonal) influenza viruses, SARS and other novel coronaviruses, smallpox, filoviruses, flaviviruses, or any micro-organism determined as potentially notifiable under Annex 2 of the International Health Regulations (IHR).  Additionally, this guide would apply to novel pathogens and pathogens with high rates of morbidity, mortality and/or transmissibility.

These pathogens include, but are not limited to:

### Tier 1 – respiratory pathogens

- Novel influenza viruses: multiplying the historic pandemic attack rate (24% to 38%) times the global population (~7 billion) times the case-fatality ratio (.04% to 60%) would produce an estimate of between 700,000 and 1.4 billion fatalities from a pandemic of a virulent influenza virus strain. 1918 ~2.5% case fatality rate (CFR); 2009 H1N1 0.01% and 0.04% CFR
  - H7N9 – China – 34% case fatality rate (CFR); U.S. H7N9 vaccine stockpiled (has not spread readily from person to person, but could adapt to become more transmissible between people)
  - H5N1 – Asia, Europe, Africa and the Middle East – 53% CFR; U.S. stockpile of H5N1 vaccine (has not spread readily from person to person, but could adapt to become more transmissible between people)
  - H3N2 – this is a current exception to the reporting policy because, while it is still considered to be a novel influenza virus and infections occur sporadically outside of the normal flu seasons, the virus does not spread easily from human to human. Since 2012 when the variant was first identified, infections have occurred via human contact with domestic swine, and there is limited evidence for secondary cases. H3N2 infectious could trigger additional actions if there was documented human-to-human transmission.
  - Other novel influenza viruses – H10N8, H5N6, H5N8, avian H5 viruses in North America
- Coronaviruses: MERS-CoV (reservoir: bats, camels) -18-62% CFR, SARS (reservoir: unknown) - 11-17% CFR
- Orthopox viruses: Smallpox (Variola), monkeypox

### Tier 2 – transmission via fluid contact

- Arenaviruses
  - Lassa (reservoir: multimammate rat)-1% CFR
- Filoviruses
  - Ebola (reservoir presumed to be bats, but unconfirmed) - 50% CFR West Africa 2014-2015
  - Marburg (reservoir: bats)-25% CFR
- Paramyxoviruses
  - Hendra (reservoir: bats; intermediate: horses)- 50% CFR
  - Nipah (reservoir: bats; intermediate: pigs)-74% CFR

### Tier 3 – vector transmission

- *Yersinia pestis* (pneumonic plague) –fleas from rodents (chipmunks, prairie dogs, ground squirrels, mice, and other mammals (dogs) =>human to human
  100% CFR for delayed treatment
- Arboviruses
  - Dengue, Chikungunya, Zika – primarily mosquitos

9

Table 3: Sample of pathogens and characteristics that would determine response:

| Pathogen | Primary Mode of transmission among people | Clinical Severity | Medical Countermeasures | Transport or Treat in place? | Pandemic potential |
|---|---|---|---|---|---|
| Ebola virus | Direct contact with bodily fluids of infected, contaminated surfaces | High | Some experimental | Typically transport | Low, assuming access to healthcare |
| MERS-CoV | Close contact, respiratory secretions | Can be high, especially in those with underlying conditions | No | Treat in place | Unknown |
| Influenza | Respiratory secretions, droplets, contact with contaminated surfaces | Can be high, especially naïve populations or in those with underlying conditions | Yes, but strain-specific vaccine must be produced | Treat in place | High for a novel strain adapted to humans |

## V.    Other Key Considerations

- **MCM, Deployment of Medical Personnel, and Biological Sample Sharing:** The existence and available supply of MCM is a key issue in considering the risks associated with an outbreak and the response. MCM availability and development must be prioritized at high levels of the U.S. Government and mobilized early in any emerging infectious threat incident. Additionally, planning (legal, regulatory, logistical, funding) for the deployment of prioritized MCM if available, and their development if not, must also be done early. At the onset of an emerging threat, the inclusion of HHS experts in clinical medicine and research would help to determine whether an HHS Emergency Medical Countermeasures Response Plan is needed. Existing mechanisms for this planning include the Public Health Emergency Medical Countermeasures Enterprise (PHEMCE) and the HHS International Sharing of Medical Countermeasures Policy Group. Mechanisms for the international deployment of public health, research, and medical personnel are required, such as the HHS International Policy Group for Personnel Sharing. Finally, similar measures must be considered for sharing samples of biological materials. Sharing of non-influenza samples is coordinated through the U.S. Government Sample Sharing Working Group, led by HHS.

- **Financial and Staffing Resources:** Financial and staffing resource planning, including deliberations on supplemental funding requests, to mount an infectious disease response needs to be considered in early stages with close coordination with the Office of Management and Budget. Collaboration with the host government to reduce issues of duplication and determine the best use of resources for the response is also necessary.

- **Adapting Risk Ratings:** The trigger criteria for evaluating an emerging infectious disease threat as an evolving public health emergency will require continual reassessment of the pathogen, location (urban vs. rural), epidemiology, host nation's capacity to respond, and disruption of health systems. Assessment tools to aid in determining trigger criteria are in continual development and should be frequently reviewed and utilized, as appropriate.

- **Triggers for Activating United Nations (UN) Cluster System and USAID/OFDA DART:** Additionally, we recommend early discussion to determine USAID/OFDA and UN OCHA's triggers for activation within an evolving public health emergency and whether any particular instance of a public health emergency could potentially trigger UN/OCHA or USAID/OFDA thresholds for activation of the cluster system or a DART. USAID/OFDA will communicate with USAID/GH Mission and USAID/OFDA Regional offices in order to monitor disease outbreaks with epidemic/pandemic potential in humanitarian crisis settings. Furthermore, USAID/OFDA will closely coordinate with CDC headquarters and country offices to monitor such outbreaks.

- **Coordinating Simultaneous U.S. government International and Domestic Responses:** The U.S. government international and domestic responses to evolving public health crises should be coordinated, as appropriate, through the NSC's coordination mechanisms. For example, coordinating availability and access to medical countermeasures, medical personnel, and laboratory specimens for national health security purposes should be balanced with the international assistance that U.S. may need to provide both to contain an outbreak before it reaches our borders or for humanitarian reasons. In particular, the existence and available supply of medical countermeasures is a key issue in considering the risks associated with an outbreak and the response.

- **Standardized Clinical Care:** Standardized clinical care must be informed by evidence. In the context of an emerging infectious disease threat, early clinical research will be critical to inform understanding of the pathophysiology and optimal clinical management to inform clinical care guidelines. In an international incident, U.S. departments and agencies will need to work with the host government and its Ministry of Health, WHO, and implementation partners on the consistent application of standardized clinical care guidance/protocols, once developed and adopted to various settings and through NGO, government, and UN partners. As expeditious clinical research on medical countermeasure advances, clinical care guidelines will need to be revisited.

# CHAPTER II – PLAYBOOK:

## DECISION-MAKING RUBRICS FOR RESPONSE TO INTERNATIONAL AND DOMESTIC EMERGING INFECTIOUS DISEASE THREATS

## I. International Playbook: Decision-Making Rubric for Assessment and Response

1. **Background:** Based on lessons learned from the 2014 Ebola outbreak and heightened monitoring of the MERS-CoV and Zika outbreaks that have followed, this international assistance and response checklist has been developed to identify key questions, U.S. Government interagency partners, and decisions to guide possible response measures in the event of a large scale infectious disease outbreak in a country(ies) with unmet public health capacity needs. The following Rubric lays out proposed initial interagency response steps, timelines, and key issues for consideration/decision, recognizing that each outbreak and country situation is different and departments and agencies have different capacities and presence on the ground. For example, CDC and USAID may already have a standing presence on the ground, allowing them to engage prior to a larger outbreak.

The Rubric is intended to focus on emerging infectious disease threats that would result in an immediate and vigorous public health response including, but are not limited to, novel (non-seasonal) influenza viruses when first discovered in circulation, Severe Acute Respiratory Syndrome (SARS) and other novel coronaviruses, smallpox (Variola) virus, wild-type poliovirus infectious outside of the current endemic areas. Those conditions, as well as infections caused by filoviruses, flaviviruses, or any microorganism determined to have significant potential to impact national health security and/or spread internationally are notifiable under Articles 6 or 7 of the International Health Regulations (IHR). Additionally, this Rubric would apply to novel pathogens and pathogens with high rates of morbidity, mortality and/or transmissibility.

This Rubric is not intended to serve as a comprehensive concept of operations or replace national or pre-existing U.S. Government response structures, but rather to serve as a proposed guide based on existing authorities, guidance, and response frameworks for staff monitoring emerging infectious disease threats and interagency planning and response, should the need arise in the future. This document is divided into two sections: key questions that provide the foundation for analytic work and key decisions and response options in accordance with the epidemiologic rating.

This Rubric is not intended to supplant other existing guidance such as the U.S. Government international disaster response system, United States Government International Chemical, Biological, Radiological, and Nuclear Response (ICBRNR) Protocol)[1] and the United States Government Policy Framework for Responding to International Requests for

---

[1] The ICBRNR Protocol provides principles, guidance and considerations for a U.S. Government response to a catastrophic, international CBRN incident. The protocol is designed to support, not supplant, existing U.S. Government coordination processes by adding CBRN-specific considerations including unique U.S. Government assistance and advisory options. It will also be used only when no other CBRN-related guidance is available or normal government to government support procedures cannot be applied (such as during war or when international response plans and agreements exist.)

Public Health and Medical Assistance during an Influenza Pandemic (PI Framework, see Appendix B)[2] or those of the World Health Organization and the Global Outbreak Alert & Response Network (GOARN). Users are encouraged to refer to these existing documents, as applicable.

2. **Assumptions:** This Rubric is based on the following key assumptions:

- The U.S. Government has the mandate and capacity to support outbreak and epidemic response in other countries through different departments and agencies. This Rubric is based on the existing legal authorities and mandates of the Departments and Agencies that would be involved in assistance and response efforts overseas. As such, the following departments and agencies should be consulted in an interagency process: DOS, USAID, HHS (in particular CDC, OGA, NIH, and other HHS components as needed), DOD, USDA, EPA, and DHS. A full description of department and agency roles begins on page 43. The National Security Council staff will provide the interagency forum and will recommend improvements to the existing mechanisms in place for a U.S. Government response to an epidemic and coordinate the policy aspects of the U.S. Government response as necessary.

- Each evolving epidemic threat will be different and will be evaluated along four dimensions of risk: (1) epidemiological indicators; (2) humanitarian/development/public health impact indicators; (3) security and political stability indicators; (4) and its transmission/outbreak/potential for public concern in the United States.

- Subject to overarching Chief of Mission[3] authority, the department or agency leading the response may differ based on the nature and phase of the outbreak or epidemic threat. Assessment teams should include expertise in infectious diseases, clinical research, epidemiology, humanitarian response, and other as needed. For example, the initial evaluation of an outbreak and provision of technical assistance may be through CDC with support from USAID, NIH, and/or DOD. A worsening outbreak may require the Chief of Mission to declare a disaster and mobilize OFDA resources to support response efforts and broader second-order humanitarian impacts through the deployment of a DART, specifically staffed for an epidemiologic response and which integrates USAID and CDC into a single incident

---

[2] The PI Framework outlines the interagency process by which the U.S. Government will receive, consider, communicate about, decide upon, and respond to international requests for public health and medical assistance during influenza pandemics. The PI Framework does not apply to routine seasonal influenza activities.

[3] By statute and the President's Letter of Instruction to COMs, the COM has full responsibility for the direction, coordination, and supervision of all U.S. executive branch employees in his or her country, regardless of their employment categories or location, except those under the command of a Geographic Combatant Commander (GCC), on the staff of an international organization, or Voice of America correspondents on assignment. With these exceptions, the COM is in charge of all executive branch activities and operations in his or her country. Agencies and employees under COM authority must keep the COM fully informed of all current and planned activities and comply with all applicable COM policies and directives. In addition, the COM and the GCC must keep each other currently and fully informed and cooperate on all matters of mutual interest.

command structure under the DART team leader. Additional DOD, HHS, and CDC resources can be brought to support response efforts through the DART's civilian incident/operational command. A worsening epidemic threat in the middle of a complex emergency or conflict situation may require a different incident command structure.

- U.S. Government epidemic threat assessments, offers of assistance, and response will be coordinated with the host government, WHO, UN humanitarian response actors, and other countries. Nevertheless, the U.S. Government will make independent assessments of the epidemic threat and response options, along the four tiers noted below.

> **For each section of the following decision-making rubrics, "Key Questions" are followed by "Key Decisions." The Key Questions are intended to be asked, including of the departments and agencies listed, in order to inform the Key Decisions that can be made and actions that can be taken.**

**1a. Normal Ops:** No unusual infectious disease outbreaks. Departments and Agencies are monitoring per usual systems.

**1b. Elevated Threat:** Infectious disease outbreak with high mortality or morbidity/clinical severity/public health consequences, high transmission or outbreak potential; case reports/cluster of high consequence infectious disease with limited countermeasures; case reports/ cluster of novel pathogen

| Key Questions* <br> *For each section of the rubric, Key Questions are followed by Key Decisions. The Key Questions are intended to be asked, including of the departments and agencies listed, in order to determine decisions that can be made and actions that can be taken | Department/Agency Responsibility | Notes |
|---|---|---|
| **Epidemiology and Country Context** <br> • What are the disease characteristics, i.e., severity, transmission potential? <br> • What is known about the current epidemiology, i.e., index case, cases, contacts? <br> • Does the host country have local diagnostic capability, contact tracing capability? <br> • Does the host country have capability to prevent, rapidly treat, and deliver medical interventions? | • **HHS (CDC, ASPR, NIH, plus others), USAID, STATE, USDA** | Note: The epidemiologic analysis and country context is important to gauge the severity of the outbreak, host country capacity to respond and whether there are known evidence-based public health interventions. <br><br> NOTE: DOD's Armed Forces Health Surveillance Center and National Center for Medical Intelligence also answers these questions specifically for DOD |

| | | |
|---|---|---|
| • Does the host country have in place the plans and capacity to implement non-pharmaceutical interventions and public health recommendations?<br>• Does the host country have communications capability to the international community through IHR channels?<br>• Does the host country have internal risk communications capability to effectively implement public health recommendations? | | |
| **Public Health Infrastructure**<br>• How strong is the host country's public health infrastructure?<br>• Has the host country undergone a Joint External Evaluation and are the results available?<br>• Does the host country have the capacity to conduct a research agenda?<br>• How strong is the country's risk communication capability | • **HHS (CDC, NIH, ASPR, plus others), USAID, STATE, USDA** | Note: This analysis provides information on the strength and capacity of the host country's public health system. The JEE, if completed, will provide insight on specific areas of weakness that may need to be shored up through external assistance. |
| **Intent**<br>• Is there evidence of deliberative intent? | • **IC, DHS, State, HHS, DOD** | Note: Evidence of intent will trigger additional investigation, response, and attribution processes led by #CT and #WMD-T and require strong coordination and input from IC, DOD, State, FBI, and DHS |
| **Specimen Sharing**<br>• Do we have access to/are we able to share among U.S. Government partners biological samples for purposes of risk assessment, research, MCM R&D, etc. | • **HHS (ASPR, CDC, and others)** | Note: Specimen sharing is critical to accelerate the development of needed countermeasures i.e. diagnostics, vaccines, and therapeutics |
| **WHO and other regional partners**<br>• What is the WHO, host country, and/or regional capacity to coordinate an operational response?<br>• Is there another donor nation or regional organization (e.g. GOARN, AUD, APEC, OAS, etc.) that has a leading role in any response due to the relationship with the host country's government? | • **State, USAID, HHS (CDC, ASPR, plus others)** | Note: WHO country offices will often play a leadership and advisor role to Ministries of Health in an outbreak. It is important to note that WHO's coordination capacity and leadership across countries varies greatly and can impact the speed of outbreak response. |
| **U.S. Bilateral Relationships**<br>• How strong are the U.S. Government and other bilateral diplomatic relationships?<br>• Is there a USAID, CDC, USDA, HHS, or DOD presence on the ground, with appropriate authorities, and who is best positioned to be a technical interlocutor with Ministry of Health? | • **STATE, USAID, HHS (CDC, ASPR, OGA), DOD, USDA** | Note: U.S. government relationship with the host government will impact the US ability to provide assistance, obtain important public health data, and/or cooperate on outbreak issues. |

| | | |
|---|---|---|
| • What additional Ministries should the U.S. Government maintain close engagement with? | | |
| **Protection of U.S. Persons and Forces Overseas**<br>• Are there U.S. Persons/Forces who are cases or contacts?<br>• Are there U.S. Persons/Force health protection concerns?<br>• What is the plan to care for U.S. civilians in the affected host country? Military personnel and other U.S. Government representatives? When might medevac/repatriation be considered? | • **STATE, DOD, DOL, HHS CDC, ASPR, and others)** | Note: DOD and State may make different assessments with respect to public health measures for U.S. forces versus U.S. persons, including Embassy staff. While it is optimal that DOD and State harmonize public health measures for both U.S. forces and U.S. persons overseas, there may be legitimate extenuating circumstances that lead DOD to take stricter quarantine and isolation measures for U.S. forces. |
| **Border Screening**<br>• Can the disease be effectively screened in travelers as a means to stop transmission?<br>• Is the disease/outbreak amenable to screening? Are there overt observable signs of illness?<br>• What is the geographical distribution of cases from the outbreak? If the outbreak covers a large area, then there are often not enough control points to implement effective border measures. If the outbreak is in a region that has a large volume of travel, then screening all travelers from that region becomes operationally difficult, if not impossible<br>• Are travel or screening and monitoring requirements either globally or at U.S. borders, appropriate and would those measures stop the spread of disease | • **HHS (including CDC, ASPR), DHS, DOL, DOT, and State** | Note: The issue of border screening is complex and requires legal and operational consultations and a public health determination on its value as a tool to slow the spread of diseases vis a vis harm to travel, trade, and ability to mount a response within affected region. It is rarely appropriate to put border screening measures in place at an elevated threat level. There needs to be close coordination with appropriate NSC staff and DHS on these issues. |
| **Key Decisions***<br>*For each section of the rubric, Key Questions are followed by Key Decisions. The Key Decisions are intended to be informed by the Key Questions listed above.* | **Department/Agency Responsibility** | **Notes** |
| • Sub-IPC/IPC to recommend overall posture: Monitor, Conduct Deeper Assessment; or Offer Technical Assistance (Advisory)<br><br>• Determine joint reporting structure and frequency of situation reports | • Sub-IPC/IPC<br><br><br>• Sub-IPC/IPC | Note: We recommend regular re-assessment or these decisions at the sub-IPC/IPC level based on the evolving situation. |

18

| | | |
|---|---|---|
| • Determine the need for and coordination of U.S. Government offers of technical advice/assistance | • **STATE, USAID, HHS (CDC, OGA, NIH, ASPR and others), USDA** | |
| • Determine whether to issue travel/ health advisory | • **STATE and CDC** | |
| • Determine the need for higher level engagement on research and development of countermeasures | • **HHS (NIH, CDC, ASPR/BARDA, OPP, FDA)** | |
| • Determine the risk communication strategy (this should be included in the travel/health advisory decision) | • **STATE** | |

**1c.  Credible Threat:**  Infectious disease outbreak with high mortality/clinical severity/high transmission; infectious disease outbreak with limited countermeasures; novel pathogen; community transmission; rate of transmission is higher than average rates/number of cases above prior outbreak thresholds; case imported to the U.S. regardless of evidence of community transmission.

| Key Questions | Department/Agency Responsibility | Notes |
|---|---|---|
| **Epidemiology and Country Context**<br>• What is the rate of transmission and projections for number of cases?<br>• Is the disease exhibiting different characteristics in terms of rate of transmission, clinical severity, etc.?<br>• What is our level of confidence on the case detection rate?<br>• Is the host government being transparent with data sharing?<br>• What is WHO's assessment?<br>• What is U.S. Government's assessment of WHO (or regional agencies) leadership in the host country?<br>• If relevant, what is the robustness of contact tracing?<br>• Is diagnostic capacity keeping up?<br>• What is our assessment of the strength of control measures?<br>• Is the public health infrastructure keeping up with the cases?  Future assessment of capacity, based on epi projection? | • **HHS (CDC, NIH plus others), USAID, STATE, USDA** | Note:  These questions are intended to build on the questions that were raised in the previous phase. At this phase, regular communication and exchange of information through sub-IPC, IPC or interagency synch process is recommended<br><br>Note:  The epidemiologic analysis and country context is important to gauge the severity of the outbreak, host country capacity to respond and whether there are known evidence-based public health interventions.<br><br>Note:  DOD's AFHSB and NCMI also answer these questions specifically for DOD |

| | | |
|---|---|---|
| **Public Health Infrastructure**<br>• How strong is the host country's public health infrastructure?<br>• Has the host country undergone a Joint External Evaluation and are the results available?<br>• Does the host country have the capacity to conduct a research agenda? | • **HHS (CDC, ASPR, plus others), USAID, STATE, USDA** | Note: This analysis provides information on the strength and capacity of the host country's public health system. The JEE, if completed, will provide insight on specific areas of weakness that may need to be shored up through external assistance. |
| **Development and Humanitarian Impacts**<br>• What is the potential for secondary impacts i.e. food security due to quarantines, orphans, etc.?<br>• What is the host country's government communication capability and public's reaction to date? | • **USAID, STATE, HHS (CDC and others)** | Note: This analysis is critical to assess secondary humanitarian, development, and economic impacts that may emerge from a growing public health crisis including: trade, migration, loss of life, livelihood, famine, and orphans/vulnerable children |
| **Countermeasures and Clinical Care**<br>• Is clinical guidance available and agreed to among the experts, including in low resource settings?<br>• Is quality clinical care available that is appropriate to standards of care in the existing setting?<br>• Is it scalable from within the region, if number of cases grow? i.e. number of clinical staff, number of beds, with additional surge capacity. In addition, triage capacity at the level of health facilities needs to be assessed as this can potential y lead to nosocomial infections.<br>• Are there surge mechanisms in place for supply chain to accommodate additional cases?<br>• Are there countermeasures, such as treatments, or vaccines currently available or under development? If so, would the affected country have access to them or would need US support?<br>• What U.S. sponsored research and development efforts are underway?<br>• Should efforts be accelerated? | • **HHS (CDC, NIH, ASPR/BARDA, OPP, FDA), USAID, DOD, USDA** | Note: This analysis is critical to inform the medical clinical response, protection of health care workers, deployment of medical countermeasures and options to stem the outbreak, loss of life and other clinical effects. |
| **Protection of U.S. Persons and Forces Overseas**<br>• Are there U.S. Persons/Forces who are cases or contacts?<br>• Are there U.S. Persons/Force health protection concerns?<br>• What is the plan to care for U.S. civilians in the affected country? Military personnel and other U.S. Government representatives? | • **STATE/DOD/(HHS including CDC, ASPR and others)** | Note: DOD and State may make different assessments with respect to public health measures for U.S. forces versus U.S. persons, including Embassy staff. While it is optimal that DOD and State harmonize public health measures for both U.S. forces and U.S. persons |

| | | |
|---|---|---|
| When might medevac/ repatriation be considered? U.S. persons or forces? | | overseas, we note in the past, there were legitimate extenuating circumstances which led DOD to take stricter quarantine and isolation measures for U.S. forces. |
| **Political/Security Analysis**<br>• What is the overall assessment of the host country's government handling of the situation?<br>• Are there any political or security overlays or implications? | • **STATE/IC/DOD** | Note: This analysis is important to assess the current and potential impact a growing public health crisis could have on political and regional security and stability. A government's mishandling of the public health crisis and rising panic could lead to instability or insecurity. |
| **U.S. Government Assistance**<br>• Is the cooperation and information sharing between the host country's government and US interlocutors strong?<br>• Has a disaster declaration been issued?<br>• Is there openness to accepting international and/or U.S. assistance? | • **STATE/USAID/HHS (including CDC, OGA, others)** | Note: U.S. Government relationship with the host government will impact the US ability to provide assistance, obtain important public health data, and/or cooperate on outbreak issues. Depending on the severity of the outbreak and secondary impact, the Chief of Mission could issue a Disaster Declaration to formerly trigger USAID's Office of Foreign Disasters funding and response mechanisms. |
| **Border Screening**<br>• Can the disease be effectively screened in travelers as a means to stop transmission?<br>• Is the disease/outbreak amenable to screening? Are there overt observable signs of illness?<br>• What is the geographical distribution of cases from the outbreak? If the outbreak covers a large area, then there are often not enough control points to implement effective border measures. If the outbreak is in a region that has a large volume of travel, then screening all travelers from that region becomes operationally difficult, if not impossible<br>• Are travel or screening and monitoring requirements either globally or at U.S. borders, appropriate and would those measures stop the spread of disease | • **HHS (including CDC, ASPR), DHS, DOL, DOT, and State** | Note: The issue of border screening is complex and requires extensive and operational consultations and a public health determination on its value as a tool to slow the spread of diseases vis a vis harm to travel, trade, and ability to mount a response within affected region. There needs to be close coordination with #TRANSBORDER and DHS on these issues. |

21

| Key Decisions | Department/Agency Responsibility | Notes |
|---|---|---|
| • Sub-IPC/IPC to advise on overall posture: Monitor, Conduct Deeper Assessment; or Offer Assistance | • Sub IPC/IPC | Note: We recommend regular re-assessment of these decisions at the sub-IPC/IPC level based on the evolving situation. |
| • Determine joint reporting structure and frequency of situation reports | • Sub IPC/IPC | |
| • Determine the need for and coordination of U.S. Government offers of technical advice/assistance. | • Sub IPC/IPC | |
| • Determine the strength of the international response, assistance from WHO, or other UN agencies, regional organizations, humanitarian systems, or other major donors. | • IPC/DC | Note: Important to assess whether WHO is providing strong leadership and press for early engagement from the international response community. |
| • Should the U.S. Government conduct an on the ground situation assessment or use existing data/reports?<br><br>   • Which Agencies should be involved—CDC, USAID/OFDA, DOD Humanitarian Assistance Support Team?<br>   • Is the environment hostile or non-permissive? | • State COM/Sub IPC/IPC | Note: Chief of Mission would need to secure host government permission to freely move around country. Decision should be made quickly and assessment team ready to go within few days. In a non-permissive environment, the US would need to rely more heavily on UN partners. |
| • Determine a full spectrum of U.S. response options and assets based on the current and potentially worsening scenarios. | • Sub IPC/IPC | Note: We recommend developing response options for worsening situations as soon as possible given the unpredictability and speed of evolving epidemics. |
| • Is there sufficient funding for the response? What are funding options? | • OMB/HHS/STATE/USAID/ DC/PC/POTUS | Note: We recommend early budget and financial analysis of various response scenarios and an early decision to request supplemental funding from Congress, if needed. |

| | | |
|---|---|---|
| • Should a Disaster Declaration and DART deployment be considered at this stage?<br>   • If yes, then what are the key lines of effort and capabilities?<br>   • If no, what are the triggers and thresholds for activating?<br>   • What support is being contemplated by the UN, WHO, key allies and like-minded countries?<br>   • Has UN OCHA determined triggers for activation? | • **State COM/USAID OFDA/IPC/DC** | Note: Foreign assistance package development should be simultaneous and informed by assessment team in real time, if there is one. Decision should be made rapidly and concurrently as assessment team is deployed and foreign assistance package is being developed. |
| • Should the U.S. begin high-level consultations on an appropriate international response? | • **IPC/DC** | Note: Discussions could occur at WHO, through GHSI, other venues. |
| • Should there be changes in Travel/ health advisory issuance? | • **State/HHS/CDC** | |
| • Should there be arrangements for medevac or in-country clinical care advisory for U.S. Persons? | • **STATE/HHS (NIH, CDC, ASPR, BARDA, FDA)** | |
| • Should there be high level engagement on research and development of countermeasures? | • **HHS (ASPR, NIH, CDC, FDA)** | |
| • Is a Public Readiness and Emergency Preparedness (PREP) Act declaration needed to support countermeasure development? | • **HHS (ASPR, HHS, NIH, CDC, FDA)** | |
| • If: the U.S. has potential countermeasures in Strategic National Stockpile (SNS), or is in the process of developing countermeasures, should any be donated in response efforts? | • **HHS (ASPR, CDC, OGA), PC** | Note: In considering deployment of SNS assets, deploying internationally in early stages may slow or prevent biological threats from reaching U.S. borders. Additionally, international needs/donations should be considered in early discussions and decisions regarding medical countermeasure research and development |
| • Determine whether to implement screening and monitoring measures, or other travel measures within the U.S. or press for measures globally | • **HHS (ASPR, CDC, OGA), PC, POTUS** | |

**2a. Public Health Emergency of International Concern (PHEIC) or PHEIC-equivalent:** An official WHO declaration of Public Health Emergency of International Concern. The term Public Health Emergency of International Concern is defined in the IHR (2005) as "an extraordinary event which is determined, as provided in these Regulations: to constitute a public health risk to other States through the international spread of disease; and to potentially require a coordinated international response". This definition implies a situation that: is serious, unusual or unexpected; carries implications for public health beyond the affected State's national border; and may require immediate international action. We recommend continuous evaluation and adjustment to the response based on whether the PHEIC is improving or worsening.

| Key Questions | Department/Agency Responsibility | Notes |
|---|---|---|
| **Epidemiology and Country Context**<br>• What is the rate of transmission and projections for number of cases?<br>• Is the disease exhibiting different characteristics in terms of rate of transmission, clinical severity, etc.?<br>• What is our level of confidence on the case detection rate?<br>• Is the host country's government being transparent with data sharing?<br>• What is WHO and/or OCHA's assessment?<br>• What is U.S. Government's assessment of OCHA and WHO leadership at the regional and host country level?<br>• If relevant, what is the robustness of contact tracing?<br>• Is diagnostic capacity keeping up?<br>• What is our assessment of the strength of the host country's control measures?<br>• Has the disease spread to other countries? | • HHS (CDC, NIH, plus others), USAID, STATE, USDA | Note: These questions are intended to build on and revisit the questions that were raised in the previous phase. At this phase, regular communication and exchange of information through sub-IPC or IPC interagency synch process is recommended; in addition to regular meetings at the Deputies level to provide guidance to Departments and Agencies and continuously evaluate the effectiveness of the response.<br><br>Note: The epidemiologic analysis and country context is likely to be dynamic and change. We recommend continuous reevaluation of the epidemiology to inform changes in US response options. |
| **Public Health Infrastructure**<br>• Is the host country's public health infrastructure overwhelmed? Assessment of future capacity, based on epi projection? | • HHS (CDC, ASPR, plus others), USAID, STATE, USDA | Note: The host country's public health infrastructure requires continuous reevaluation of the epidemiology to ensure that diagnostic and medical care capacity is keeping up with the needs. |
| **Humanitarian and Development Impacts**<br>• What is the potential for secondary impacts i.e. food security due to quarantines, orphans, etc.? | • USAID, STATE | Note: The humanitarian impact is likely to change and worsen as the public health crisis worsens. The U.S. should assess the need to layer in other humanitarian interventions |

| | | |
|---|---|---|
| • What is the host country's government communication capability and public's reaction to date? | | (food; water, sanitation, and hygiene; shelter) and whether to press for activation of the UN OCHA cluster system. |
| **Countermeasures and Clinical Care**<br>• Is clinical guidance available and agreed to among the experts, including in low resource settings?<br>• Is quality clinical care available in the existing setting?<br>• Is clinical care capacity scalable, if number of cases grow?<br>• Is it scalable from within the region, if number of cases grow? i.e. number of clinical staff, number of beds, with additional surge capacity. In addition, triage capacity at the level of health facilities needs to be assessed as this can potentially lead to nosocomial infections.<br>• Are there surge mechanisms in place for supply chain to accommodate additional cases?<br>• Are countermeasures or vaccines currently available or under development?<br>• What US sponsored research and development efforts are underway?<br>• Should efforts be accelerated? | • **HHS (ASPR,NIH,CDC,FDA), DOD, USAID** | Note: This analysis is critical to inform whether the medical clinical response needs augmentation or protocols need adjustment to improve clinical outcomes. There may also be a need to prioritize deployment of countermeasures based on supplies and accelerate research and development. |
| **Protection of U.S. Persons and Forces Overseas**<br>• Are there U.S. Persons/Forces who are cases or contacts?<br>• Are there U.S. Persons/Force health protection concerns?<br>• What is the plan to care for U.S. civilians in the affected country? Military personnel and other U.S. Government representatives? When might medevac/repatriation be considered?<br>• U.S. persons or forces? | • **STATE, DOD, DOL, HHS** | Note: DOD and State may make different assessments with respect to public health measures for US forces versus U.S. persons, including Embassy staff. While it is optimal that DOD and State harmonize public health measures for both U.S. forces and U.S. persons overseas, there may be legitimate extenuating circumstances that lead DOD to take stricter quarantine and isolation measures for U.S. forces. |
| **Political/Security Analysis**<br>• What is the overall assessment of the host country's government handling of the situation?<br>• Are there any political or security overlays or implications? | • **STATE/IC/DOD** | Note: This analysis requires continued updating and assessment of evolving security risks. A government's mishandling of the public health crisis and rising panic could lead to instability or insecurity. |

| U.S. Government Assistance | • STATE, USAID, HHS (CDC, ASPR, OGA, others) | Note: U.S. Government relationship with the host government will impact the US ability to provide assistance, obtain important public health data, and/or cooperate on outbreak issues. Depending on the severity of the outbreak and secondary impact, the Chief of Mission could issue a Disaster Declaration to formerly trigger USAID's Office of Foreign Disasters funding and response mechanisms |
|---|---|---|
| • Is the cooperation and information sharing between the host country's government and US interlocutors strong?<br>• Has a disaster declaration been issued?<br>• Is there openness to accepting international and/or US assistance?<br>• Is WHO or UNOCHA coordinating the response? What role do regional agencies (e.g., PAHO) have at this stage?<br>• What partners/allies do we press for assistance?<br>• Are there legal issues with the host country's government that need to be addressed with respect to provision of assistance? | | |
| **Embassy Security**<br>• What is the Embassy's overall security and operating posture i.e. authorized departures, ordered departures, advisories to US citizens, other security concerns? | • STATE | |
| **Border Screening**<br>• Can the disease be effectively screened in travelers as a means to stop transmission?<br>• Is the disease/outbreak amenable to screening? Are there overt observable signs of illness?<br>• What is the geographical distribution of cases from the outbreak? If the outbreak covers a large area, then there are often not enough control points to implement effective border measures. If the outbreak is in a region that has a large volume of travel, then screening all travelers from that region becomes operationally difficult, if not impossible<br>• Are travel or screening and monitoring requirements either globally or at U.S. borders, appropriate and would those measures stop the spread of disease | • HHS (including CDC, ASPR), DHS, DOL, DOT, and State | Note: The issue of border screening is complex and requires legal and operational consultations and a public health determination on its value as a tool to slow the spread of diseases vis a vis harm to travel, trade, and ability to mount a response within affected region. There needs to be close coordination with #TRANSBORDER and DHS on these issues. |

| **Key Decisions** | **Department/Agency Responsibility** | **Notes** |
|---|---|---|
| • Sub-IPC/IPC to advise on overall posture: Monitor; Offer Assistance; Mount Response | • Sub-IPC/IPC | Note: We recommend regular re-assessment of these decisions at the DC level based on the evolving situation. |

| | | |
|---|---|---|
| • Determine whether existing international and/or U.S. technical assistance efforts making a difference in the trajectory of the disease and if changes are needed. | • **Sub-IPC/IPC/DC** | Note: Foreign assistance package development should be simultaneous and informed by assessment team in real time, if there is one. |
| • Should a Disaster Declaration and USAID/OFDA DART deployment be considered at this stage?<br><br>    • If yes, then what are the key lines of effort and capabilities among Agencies?<br>    • If no, what are the triggers and thresholds for activating?<br>    • What support is being contemplated by the UN, WHO, key allies and like-minded countries?<br>    • Has UN OCHA determined triggers for activation? | • **State COM/USAID OFDA/IPC/DC** | Decision should be made rapidly and concurrently as assessment team is deployed and assistance package is being developed. If there is a determination that an Epi-DART deployment not needed, then triggers/threshold for mobilization should be identified as part of the DART mobilization decision, based on severity |
| • Should there be a military deployment in support of a civilian DART response? | • **DOD/USAID/STATE/DC/PC /POTUS** | Note: This option presumes that the response is primarily operated through USAID and humanitarian response community, with select limited support through DOD. As the situation warrants, especially if country health system is overwhelmed. Need to consider impacts on U.S. personnel and needs in the U.S. |
| • Should the U.S. Government provide direct patient care through Public Health Service (PHS) Commissioned Corp or DOD capabilities? | • **HHS/DOD/DC/PC/POTUS** | Note: This option may be considered as the situation warrants, especially if country health system is overwhelmed. Need to consider impacts on U.S. personnel and needs in the U.S. and will involve legal negotiations through State/L with host country on licensing of U.S. Government medical personnel. [1] Additionally, DOD's medical capability to respond to a disease outbreak is limited and untested in the field, whereas the PHS did successfully operate an Ebola Treatment Unit in Monrovia. DOD's medical system is primarily designed to triage and evacuate the sick and injured, and DOD |
| • Should the U.S. Government deploy the PHS Commissioned Corps or other public health and medical teams in support of public health efforts and response? | • **HHS/DC/PC/POTUS** | |

| | | currently has little deployable medical capability to respond to an infectious disease outbreak in another country, as our deployable capability is primarily designed for kinetic injuries. |
|---|---|---|
| • Is there sufficient funding for the response? What are funding options? | • **OMB/HHS/STATE/USAID/ DC/PC/POTUS** | Note: We recommend early budget and financial analysis of various response scenarios and an early decision to request supplemental funding from Congress, if needed. |
| • Determine travel/ health advisory issuance | • **CDC and State** | |
| • Determine whether to implement screening and monitoring measures, or other travel measures within the US or press for measures globally | • **DC/PC/POTUS** | |
| • Determine CONOP to medevac or provide in country clinical care advisory for U.S. Persons | • **STATE/HHS (including NIH, CDC, ASPR/BARDA, FDA)** | |
| • Should the U.S. mount an aggressive international diplomacy campaign to ensure the response efforts are resourced? | • **IPC/DC/PC** | Note: We recommend early high level U.S. diplomacy and requests for meaningful engagement of other countries, United Nations organizations, and multilateral institutions in order to alleviate pressure on US assets and resources and rapidly contain outbreaks before other part of the world are impacted. |
| • Should there be high level engagement on research (including non-clinical) and development of countermeasures | • **HHS (ASPR/HHS/NIH/CDC/FDA) USAID** | |

| | | |
|---|---|---|
| • Is a PREP Act declaration needed to support countermeasure/vaccine development? | • **HHS -- ASPR/HHS/NIH/CDC/FDA** | |
| • Is interagency coordination of public, diplomatic, and legislative communications necessary? | • **DC/PC** | |
| • If PHEIC is in a conflict zone where the U.S. is not already militarily engaged, should DOD be engaged in the public health response under the auspices of a lead federal agency? [4] | • **PC/NSC/POTUS** | Note: This is a complex, difficult decision and careful consideration is needed before committing the U.S. military assets in a conflict zone where the U.S. is not already militarily engaged. In particular, the decision needs consider if the risk of the disease spreading to the U.S. outweigh the security risk to U.S. personnel? What are the legal authorities for the U.S. to engage in conflict settings? Has U.S. military engagement been requested by a legitimate local authority? What are the political implications of military action? |
| • If: PHEIC is in a conflict zone where the U.S. is militarily engaged, should DOD be asked to assist with response activities in support of the Lead Federal Agency (See footnote 4)? | • **PC/NSC/POTUS** | Note: Under present authorities, DOD would be able to provide a broad spectrum of support to a response, in support of a Lead Federal Agency (i.e. USAID). Among other factors, policy makers will need to consider the impact of this support on COCOM operations vis a vis risks posed by the spread of the disease. |

---

[4] In this and the next two instances, we assume that DOD would be managing the majority of the operational response under the auspices of lead federal agency such as USAID. USAID has the delegated authority for foreign disaster assistance per E.O. 12163. Per DOD Directive 5100.46, DOD shall respond to foreign disasters in support of the U.S. Agency for International Development (USAID) pursuant to E.O. 12163 and section 2292(b) of title 22, U.S.C. In emergency situations in order to save human lives, where there is not sufficient time to seek the prior initial concurrence of the Secretary of State, in which case the Secretary of Defense shall advise, and seek the concurrence of, the Secretary of State as soon as practicable thereafter per E.O. 12966. DOD response under these circumstances is limited to 72 hours unless concurrence from the Secretary of State is received.

| | | |
|---|---|---|
| • If: in country and civilian response capabilities are completely overwhelmed with rapid airborne transmission spreading to multiple countries, should DOD support the epidemiologic response, as required, under the auspices of a Lead Federal Agency i.e. USAID (See footnote 4)? | • **PC/NSC/POTUS** | |
| • If: the U.S. has potential countermeasures in Strategic National Stockpile (SNS), or is in the process of developing countermeasures, should ary be donated in response efforts | • **HHS (ASPR, CDC, OGA), PC, POTUS** | Note: In considering deployment of SNS assets, it may be that deploying internationally in early stages may slow or prevent biological threats from reaching U.S. borders. Additionally, international needs/donations should be considered in early discussions and decisions regarding medical countermeasure research and development |

## II.    Domestic Playbook: Decision-Making Rubric for Assessment and Response

**Assumptions:**

The following assumptions will apply to an early response to a high-consequence emerging infectious disease threat in the United States:

- Early in the emergence of an emerging infectious disease threat, either within or outside the United States, there will be more that is unknown than what is known. Decision-makers will choose courses of action with incomplete information.

- The U.S. Government will use all powers at its disposal to prevent, slow, or mitigate the spread of an emerging infectious disease threat by:
    1) Limiting spread of disease;
    2) Mitigating the impact of illness, suffering, and death; and
    3) Sustaining critical infrastructure and key resources in the United States.

- The NSC will serve as an information conduit for the Executive Office of the President (EOP) and will coordinate interagency policy discussions and decisions.

- While States hold significant power and responsibility related to public health response outside of a declared Public Health Emergency, the American public will look to the U.S. Government for action when multi-state or other significant public health events occur.

- An emerging infectious disease threat could be the result of natural emergence, accident, or intentional act of terrorism. An early Federal response may include efforts to discern the cause and take appropriate action if the pathogen is found to have not emerged from nature.

| **1a. Normal Operations:** No specific threat of a pandemic. Departments and Agencies are monitoring per usual systems. |
|---|

| **1b. Elevated Threat:** Identification of a human case of a pathogen of pandemic potential (PPP) anywhere. |
|---|

| **Key Questions\*** <br> *\*For each section of the rubric, Key Questions are followed by Key Decisions. The Key Questions are intended to be asked, including of the departments and agencies listed, in order to determine decisions that can be made and actions that can be taken* | **Department/Agency Responsible** | **Notes** |
|---|---|---|
| **Epidemiology and Locality Context** <br><br> • What are the disease characteristics (i.e., severity, transmission potential) and current domestic availability of MCM, and non-pharmaceutical interventions (NPI)? <br><br> • Is the threat potential imminent or more a long-term threat? What is known about the current epidemiology (i.e. index cases, case contacts)? <br><br> • Are there clear public health or medical recommendations for prevention, treatment or other intervention sufficient to prevent an outbreak? <br><br> • Does the State, Local, Territorial, or Tribal (SLTT) jurisdiction have internal and external communication strategies and capabilities to effectively implement public service messaging? <br><br> • Does the SLTT jurisdiction have diagnostic capability and capacity sufficient to trace and monitor for an outbreak? <br><br> • Does the SLTT jurisdiction have in place the plans, capability, and capacity to implement MCM or NPI sufficient to prevent an outbreak? <br><br> • Is the disease treatable locally or does it need treatment requiring transport of patients to a specialty treatment facility? <br><br> • Will infectious waste disposal require Comprehensive Environmental Response, Compensation, and Liability Act offsite disposal and/or come under Hazardous material regulations? | • HHS <br> • FEMA <br> • EPA | HHS is the lead federal department/agency (LFA) for domestic *health response* and coordinates all other federal departments and agencies through a unified coordination structure scalable to the event. <br><br> FBI would be the LFA for law enforcement *crisis management response*. Evidence of intent will trigger additional processes and involve NSC, IC, DOD, State, FBI, DHS, and HHS. Refer to the BIA for specific interagency coordination. <br><br> The *health response* and law enforcement *crisis management response* should occur synchronously. <br><br> Refer to Planning Guidance for the Handling of Solid Waste Contaminated with a Category A Infectious Disease Substance |

| | | |
|---|---|---|
| • Are there chemical or physical tools and infrastructure sufficient to interrupt or impede transmission? | | |
| **Intent** <br> • Is there evidence of deliberate intent? | • FBI | |

| **Key Decisions*** <br> *For each section of the rubric, Key Questions are followed by Key Decisions. The Key Decisions are intended to be informed by the Key Questions listed above.* | **Department/Agency Responsible** | **Notes** |
|---|---|---|
| • Provide federal support to SLTT preparation where gaps exist. <br> • Determine the need for research and development or procurement of medical and non-MCM. <br> • Plan and prepare for federal action should threat become credible. <br> • Develop communication strategies and identify a trusted credible authority as spokesperson. <br> • Tailor waste management plans to incident specific conditions. | • HHS <br> • FBI <br> • DOT <br> • EPA | Refer to Planning Guidance for the Handling of Solid Waste Contaminated with a Category A Infectious Disease Substance |

## 1c. Credible Threat: Confirmation of multiple human cases of a PPP anywhere OR determination of a significant potential for a Public Health Emergency (PHE).

| **Key Questions** | **Department/Agency Responsible** | **Notes** |
|---|---|---|
| **Epidemiology** <br> • What is the rate of transmission and projection for number of cases? <br> • Is the disease exhibiting different characteristics in terms of rate of transmission, clinical severity, etc.? <br> • Is appropriate active surveillance underway and what is our level of confidence on the case detection rate? <br> • Are there immediate risks to the public that must be addressed or immediate actions that must take place to contain the cases? | • HHS (CDC, plus others), USDA | These questions are intended to build on the questions that were raised in the previous phase. At this phase, regular communication and exchange of information through sub-IPC, IPC or interagency synch process such as the Biological Incident Notification and Assessment (BINA) Protocol is recommended |

| | | |
|---|---|---|
| • To what extent has quarantine and isolation been implemented by local medical and public health authorities?<br>• What is the robustness of contact tracing?<br>• Is diagnostic capacity keeping up, and are the results available in a timely manner?<br>• What is our assessment of the strength of control measures?<br>• Is the public health infrastructure keeping up with the cases? Future assessment of capacity, based on epidemiologic projection?<br>• Is there specific concern for federal workforce safety?<br>• Is this pathogen susceptible to detection by screening travelers? | | |
| **Countermeasures and Clinical Care**<br>• Is clinical guidance available and agreed to among the experts, including in low resource settings?<br>• Is clinical care available at an appropriate standards of care in the existing setting?<br>• Is clinical care scalable from within the region, if number of cases grow?<br>• Are there countermeasures, such as treatments, or vaccines currently available or under development?<br>• What research and development efforts are underway?<br>• Should efforts be accelerated? | • HHS (including CDC, NIH, ASPR/BARDA, FDA), DOD, USDA | |
| **Political/Security Analysis**<br>• What is the overall assessment of the SLTT government's handling of the situation?<br>• Are there any political or security overlays or implications? | • HHS, DHS<br>• Sub-IPC | |
| **U.S. Government Assistance**<br>• Has a disaster declaration been considered? If not, what are the triggers?<br>• Is there a need to coordinate response beyond local capability?<br>• Is there a need for a United Coordination Group and if so, at what level and where to physically locate it? | • HHS, DHS | Declaration of Stafford Emergency or PHE allows funding and response and recovery resources from the Fed Gov. |

| Key Decisions | Department/Agency Responsible | Notes |
|---|---|---|
| <ul><li>Biological Incident Notification and Assessment (BINA) Protocol to engage the interagency for awareness</li><li>Sub-IPC/IPC to recommend overall posture: monitors, conduct deeper assessment; or offer technical assistance (advisory)</li><li>Determine reporting structure and frequency of situation reports</li><li>Determine the need for and coordination of federal advice/assistance.</li><li>Establish the formal structure of the UCG once determination is made to stand one up or what the triggers will be to stand one up.</li><li>Determine funding sources for a response. What are funding options?</li><li>Consider a PHE at this stage.<ul><li>If yes, identify the key lines of effort and capabilities the PHE will address.</li><li>If no, identify the triggers and thresholds for activating.</li><li>Identify all support being contemplated by the U.S. Government?</li></ul></li><li>Consider implementation of travel restrictions and border controls.</li><li>Consider the potential for changes in Travel/ health advisory issuance.</li><li>Engage on research, development, increased production of MCM or NPI if necessary.</li><li>Determine whether a PREP Act declaration needed to support MCM development.</li></ul> | <ul><li>Sub-IPC/IPC</li><li>HHS</li><li>DOT</li></ul> | Depending on the nature and predicted evolution of the threat, this could easily demand a review at the Deputies level or above. |

| 2a. Initial Response-Activation, Situational Assessment, and Movement:  Demonstration of efficient and sustained human-to-human transmission of a novel or re-emerging PPP anywhere OR Declaration of a PHE. | | |
|---|---|---|
| **Key Questions** | **Department/Agency Responsible** | **Notes** |
| **Incident Detection and Threat Characterization**<br>• What is the rate of transmission and projections for number of cases?<br>• Is the disease exhibiting different characteristics in terms of rate of transmission, clinical severity, etc.?<br>• What is our level of confidence on the case detection rate?<br>• Is the SLTT Government being transparent with data sharing?<br>• What is the robustness of contact tracing?<br>• Is diagnostic capacity keeping up? | • HHS<br>• Sub-IPC | All previous questions should be revisited at each of these response phases (2 a,b,c) in addition to those that follow.<br><br>In a rapidly evolving incident, all subsequent questions and decisions may be on the table early. |
| **Communications**<br>• What is the SLTT government's communication capability and public's reaction to date?<br>• Is U.S. Government coordinating risk communication to develop a unified message across a range of media?<br>• What are key Federal messages?<br>• Who should act as the key Federal spokesperson for the response? | • HHS (ASPA), DHS (JIC)<br>• Sub-IPC | Early coordination of risk communications through a single federal spokesperson is critical to collect and disseminate data elements from across SLTT and federal agencies. |
| **Controlling the Spread/Epidemic**<br>• Has the disease spread to other localities?<br>• What is our assessment of the strength of control measures?<br>• Is the SLTT public health infrastructure overwhelmed? Assessment of future capacity, based on epi projection?<br>• Is this going to be a Stafford Act incident (Pres)? Public Health Emergency (HHS)? Both? | • HHS/FEMA<br>• Sub-IPC | Stafford Act Incident: Participant Agencies provide support to NRF and NDRF elements (JFO, NOC, etc).  FEMA is primary for federal operations although may not be LFA.<br>Non-Stafford Act Incident: must establish alternate legal authorities of each participant for provided support activities. Support between agencies is governed by Economy Act. |

| Key Decisions | Department/Agency Responsible | Notes |
|---|---|---|
| • Determine the need for public health support personnel, teams, etc.<br>• Determine the need for diagnostic personnel teams and resources.<br>• Determine patient movement needs and methodology between designated facilities, locations, and jurisdiction.<br>• Prepare public messaging and steps the public should take to protect itself. Unify messaging with SLTT.<br>• Coordination of workforce protection activities, including threat messaging; PPE determination, procurement and deployment; compliance with OSHA requirements; development and dissemination of worker safety and health guidance (OSHA and National Institute for Occupational Safety and Health (NIOSH)); identification and clarification of workplace policies and flexibilities (Office of Personnel Management, Equal Employment Opportunity Commission).<br>• Determine regulatory approaches to facilitate MCM or NPI in the event they are needed. Emergency Use Authorizations (EUA) if novel. | • IPC/DC<br>• HHS, DHS, DOL/OSHA, NIOSH | Unified coordination (UCG) at the federal level, HHS REC coordinates with FEMA Regional Administrator |

**2b. Employment of Resources and Stabilization:** Increasing number of cases in the United States or healthcare system burden that exceeds State, Local, Territorial, or Tribal (SLTT) resources OR SLTT request of assistance.

| Key Questions | Department/Agency Responsible | Notes |
|---|---|---|
| • Is there sufficient funding for the response? What are funding options?<br>• Should a Disaster Declaration be considered at this stage?<br>  • If yes, then what are the key lines of effort and capabilities?<br>  • If no, what are the triggers and thresholds for activating?<br>  • What federal support is being contemplated? | • HHS/DHS<br>• IPC/DC | National-level UCG established with a Federal Health Coordinating Officer designated for affected states |

| Key Decisions | Department/Agency Responsible | Notes |
|---|---|---|
| • Determine whether to implement screening and monitoring measures, or other travel measures within the US or globally.<br>• Determine whether Strategic National Stockpile (SNS) resources are necessary<br>• Prioritization and allocation of resources subject to the Defense Production Act (DPA)<br>• Determine need for EUA<br>• Determine need for private sector funding and methods to establish new MCM<br>• Determine need for medical providers<br>• Determine need for mortuary services | • IPC/DC<br>• HHS<br>• DOT | |

**2c. Intermediate Operations:** Cases continue to climb with long-term service disruption and critical infrastructure impact OR Presidential Stafford Act Declaration OR SLTT request for assistance.

| Key Questions | Department/Agency Responsible | Notes |
|---|---|---|
| **Mass Care and Human Services**<br>• Does local SLTT authority need assistance to implement mass care activities such as shelter, commodity distribution or medical services?<br>• Is the incident likely to impact housing such that alternate housing needs may become necessary?<br>• Are there voluntary organizations that can be integrated into response? | • HHS, DHS<br>• IPC/DC | |
| **Augment and Surge Public Health and Medical Services**<br>• Should the U.S. Government deploy the PHS Commissioned Corps or other public health and medical teams in support of public health efforts and response? | • HHS<br>• IPC/DC/PC | |
| **Political/Security Analysis**<br>• What is the overall assessment of the government's handling of the situation?<br>• Are there any political or security overlays or implications? | • IPC/DC | |

| Border Screening<br>• Can the disease be effectively screened in travelers as a means to stop transmission?<br>• Are travel or screening and monitoring requirements either globally or at U.S. borders, appropriate and would those measures stop the spread of disease? | • HHS, DHS, DOS, DOL , DOT | The issue of border screening is very complex and requires extensive legal consultations and a public health determination on its value as a tool to slow the spread of diseases vis a vis harm to travel, trade, and ability to mount a response within affected region. There needs to be close coordination with #TRANSBORDER and DHS on these issues. |
|---|---|---|
| **Key Decisions** | **Department/Agency Responsible** | **Notes** |
| • IPC to advise on overall posture: Monitor; Offer Assistance; Mount Response<br>• Determine travel/ health advisory issuance<br>• Determine whether to implement screening and monitoring measures, or other travel measures within the US or press for measures globally.<br>• Is interagency coordination of public, diplomatic, and legislative communications necessary? | • IPC/DC/PC | |

**3a. Sustained Operations:** Long-term recovery operations with or without continued incidence of new cases.

| **Key Questions** | **Department/Agency Responsible** | **Notes** |
|---|---|---|
| • Protect, Augment, and Return Federal and SLTT Essential Services<br>• Support SLTT officials in decision-making and implementation of relocation, alternative housing, and re-occupancy strategies.  Large displaced populations will need to be linked integrally to remediation planning.<br>• What are the key services and critical infrastructure that need to come back online for society to return to normal?<br>• What Federal programs can be leveraged to assist with recovery? | • IPC/DC/PC | |

| Key Decisions | Department/Agency Responsible | Notes |
|---|---|---|
| • Emergency supplemental for recovery?<br>• National prioritization for recovery (i.e. infrastructure and schools). | • IPC/DC/PC | |

# CHAPTER III – APPENDICES

# APPENDIX

## I.  Declarations and Mitigation Options

### DECLARATIONS

There are a variety of declarations that enable the use of different governmental response authorities and activities. Described below are declarations and their authorities that would likely be considered early in a response to a pathogen with the potential to cause an epidemic emergency or a pandemic.

*WHO Declaration of Public Health Emergency of International Concern (PHEIC) (**WHO Director General**)*

A PHEIC is declared in response to an extraordinary event that is determined to constitute a public health risk through the international spread of disease, potentially requiring a coordinated international response. A PHEIC would trigger release of emergency "temporary" recommendations by the WHO regarding travel, surveillance, infection control, and medical care to affected or other countries.

*Public Health Emergency (PHE) (**HHS Secretary**)*

Under Section 319 of the Public Health Service Act, the HHS Secretary may determine that a disease or disorder presents a public health emergency or that a public health emergency, including significant outbreaks of infectious disease or bioterrorist attacks, otherwise exists. A declaration lasts for the duration of the emergency or for 90 days, and can be extended. As amended under the Pandemic and All Hazards Preparedness Reauthorization Act, a PHE enables HHS to access "no year" funds, and allows for various exemptions and waivers to facilitate response activities, including certain restrictions on requirements for medical countermeasure distribution, some Select Agent requirements. It also allows the Secretary, upon request by a governor or tribal organization, to authorize the temporary reassignment of state and local public health department or agency personnel funded in whole or in part through programs authorized under the Public Health Service Act for the purpose of immediately addressing a federally declared public health emergency.

*Presidential Declaration of a National Emergency (**POTUS**)*

The National Emergencies Act, Section 201, authorizes the President to declare a national emergency. Under Section 301, The President must specify the provisions of the law under which the President or other officials will act before statutory emergency authorities can be exercised. A declaration under the National Emergencies Act triggers emergency authorities contained in other statutes.

*Robert T. Stafford Disaster Relief and Emergency Assistance Act (POTUS)*

The President may declare an emergency under the Stafford Act (42 USC Chapter 68) when Federal assistance is needed to supplement State and local efforts and capabilities to save lives, protect property, and preserve public health and safety. The President can also declare an emergency without a gubernatorial request if primary responsibility for response rests with the Federal Government because the emergency involves a subject area for which the United States exercises exclusive responsibility and authority. This authority is less likely to be used during a health-related emergency, but FEMA has provided guidance under what conditions it could be used to enable State response efforts in an influenza pandemic.

*Social Security Act Section 1135*

Under Section 1135 of the Social Security Act the HHS Secretary is authorized to temporarily modify or waive certain Medicare, Medicaid, State Children's Health Insurance (SCHIP) programs, and waive some Health Insurance Portability and Accountability Act requirements in order to ensure sufficient healthcare services for those enrolled in SSA programs during an emergency. Section 1135 waivers require a declaration of national emergency or disaster by the POTUS under the National Emergencies Act or Stafford Act and a Public Health Emergency determination by the HHS Secretary.

## PHARMACEUTICAL/MEDICAL MITIGATION OPTIONS

Depending on the pathogen and its primary mode of transmission, there may be a series of early decisions, led by HHS, related to MCM – vaccines, drugs and other therapies to treat and prevent disease. Given that information about the nature and spread of the disease may not be readily available, these decisions may need to be made in an uncertain environment characterized by the absence of concrete and reliable information.

Key questions:

- Are there ways (such as diagnostic devices) to detect this pathogen/disease?
- What medical materiel are necessary to treat this disease?
- What supplies are needed to protect healthcare workers, others who may be in contact with patients?
- How will we address requests for international sharing of MCM?

**Are there licensed vaccines available for this threat?**

If YES: Is there vaccine held in Federal stockpiles?

If NO: Should the United States initiate purchase of vaccine?

If NO: Are there vaccines in investigational stages of development?

If YES: Should investigational vaccines be pursued for potential use?

## Are there approved drugs or other treatment options available?

If YES: Are there treatment options held in Federal stockpiles?

If NO: Should the United States purchase available drugs?
If YES: Are the treatment options available in the quantity needed?

If NO: are there treatment options in investigational stages of development?

If YES: Should investigational treatment options be pursued for potential use?

## Is there sufficient personal protective equipment for healthcare workers who are providing medical care?

If YES: What are the triggers to signal exhaustion of supplies? Are additional supplies available?

If NO: Should the Strategic National Stockpile release PPE to States?

## NON- PHARMACEUTICAL INTERVENTIONS

*Travel-related Interventions*

There are a series of potential travel-related interventions to slow or stop the spread of an emerging disease to the United States, including.

a. Working with affected countries to place restrictions on travelers exiting the impacted country(ies);
b. Working with transit countries to place restrictions on travelers coming to the United States from an affected country;
c. Providing health-related guidance to travelers entering the United States;
d. Issuing security directives or emergency amendments to place restrictions on flights entering or operating in the United States;
e. Support for the country of outbreak in containing the pathogen
f. Restricting the arrival of conveyances or individuals from affected country(ies);
g. Screening for illness at ports of entry and monitoring of potentially exposed persons; and
h. Measures such as health guidance, isolating ill passengers and/or placing exposed passengers under quarantine to limit onward disease transmission.
i. Redirection and consolidation of resources as necessary.

Key Questions:

## What is the scope of the travelling population of concern?

a) What is the volume of inbound airline passenger traffic per day, by airport of arrival, via direct and indirect travel? (DHS/CBP)
b) Are nationals of the affected country subject to visa requirements, or do they travel Visa Waiver? (State)
c) What is the size and makeup of the U.S.-persons population in the affected country? (State & DOD)

## Can the host country identify the infected and trace their contacts?

If YES:

a) Can and will the host country quarantine and isolate effectively? (HHS/CDC)
b) Can and will the host country implement effective "do not board" orders for those identified? (State & DHS)
c) Will the host country share the DNB data with the U.S. Government? (State & DHS)

If NO:

a) Are there readily detectable signs/symptoms for which we can screen? (HHS)
b) Can a population be determined for screening? (DHS, HHS/CDC, & State)
c) Can they be funneled? (DHS & DOT)

## Options other than screening:

a) United States Government- generated "do not board" lists
b) Issuance of Security Directives (domestic carriers)
c) Issuance of Emergency Amendments (foreign carriers)

## COMMUNITY MITIGATION MEASURES

Non-pharmaceutical measures are critical components of early response to an emerging epidemic or pandemic. They work best when complementing pharmaceutical interventions such as the provision of vaccines and drugs, but may be the only intervention possible when pharmaceutical options are not available. Community mitigation measures can include:

a. Voluntary home isolation of the ill and home quarantine of the exposed
b. Dismissal of students from schools
c. Social distancing measures, such as telework
d. Cancellation of large public gatherings; and
e. Widespread use of personal protective devices

## II.    Key Departments and Agencies:

### i.    International

This Rubric is based on the existing legal authorities and mandates of the Departments and Agencies that would be involved in assistance and response efforts overseas. As such, the following Departments and Agencies should be consulted in an interagency process:

- **The Department of State**: State will retain Chief of Mission authority and may facilitate requests of assistance from the host government, issue disaster declarations, and maintain high level communications.

  - **The Department of State (Embassies)**: State supports Embassy operations under Chief of Mission authority[5] in affected countries to: facilitate requests of assistance from the host government as well as encouraging host government to take effective and medically sound response measures; maintain liaison with international organizations, other donor countries, and NGOs working in the response; issue disaster declarations in consultation with USAID; maintain secure, high-level communications; provide the logistics and administrative support for U.S. personnel arriving to assist; and provide big-picture reporting on events in country.

  - **The Department of State (Headquarters)**: State reaches out to other donor countries and organization to understand existing commitments and, where appropriate, encourage additional or new commitments of resources for a response; ensures other U.S. agencies participating in the response are coordinating with Embassy and other responders, and that they have any needed bilateral agreements required for the response with host countries; communicates with other countries on matters important to response such as overflight rights, medical evacuation and treatment options; and works with HHS on diplomatic engagement with WHO, health ministers, and similar offices and officials etc.

---

[5] By statute and the President's Letter of Instruction to COMs, the COM has full responsibility for the direction, coordination, and supervision of all U.S. executive branch employees in his or her country, regardless of their employment categories or location, except those under the command of a Geographic Combatant Commander (GCC), on the staff of an international organization, or Voice of America correspondents on assignment. With these exceptions, the COM is in charge of all executive branch activities and operations in his or her country. Agencies and employees under COM authority must keep the COM fully informed of all current and planned activities and comply with all applicable COM policies and directives. In addition, the COM and the GCC must keep each other currently and fully informed and cooperate on all matters of mutual interest.

- **The United States Agency for International Development (USAID)**: USAID's Bureau for Global Health (USAID/GH) and USAID/OFDA's ongoing health, development and disaster risk reduction programs in developing countries may provide a platform for support at the request of the host government. In the event of a humanitarian emergency, USAID/OFDA coordinates operational response efforts among U.S government actors, serves as the interlocutor with the international humanitarian system, and engages with other humanitarian donors regarding resource support. USAID/OFDA will provide support to assess the humanitarian aspects of an evolving epidemic threat and may be activated to provide varying degrees of response support (case management, coordination, logistics and social mobilization) in the event of large scale public health emergency. USAID/OFDA maintains engagement in humanitarian global health networks and the international humanitarian architecture; and can also leverage partners' experience, including the UN Office for the Coordination of Humanitarian Affairs (OCHA), which coordinates UN agencies involved in humanitarian response, and international NGOs that provide medical and health services. USAID/OFDA, CDC, and DOD have existing interagency agreements that cover joint operations, exchanges of technical advisors, staff and liaison officers, and cross trainings. USAID/GH's ongoing health and development programs in developing countries may provide a platform for support at the request of the host government. Additionally, USAID/GH and USAID/OFDA, in coordination with HHS, can support diplomatic engagements with WHO. In the event of an epidemic reaching humanitarian scale, USAID/OFDA can also support U.S. Government coordination with WHO through engagements with the Health Cluster.

  USAID maintains substantial operational and technical capacities to lead overseas disaster responses, including interagency partnerships, planning, programming, logistics, sectoral expertise, and coordination. These capabilities can be mobilized toward a public health crisis when the situation occurs amidst a wider humanitarian emergency, or the health crisis constitutes a disaster in its own right. When crises require a large scale operational response, USAID deploys a Disaster Assistance Response Team (DART) to coordinate the U.S. Government interagency response. The DART is an adaptable, scalable and flexible response and coordination structure, linking major roles, responsibilities and actions of the U.S. Government efforts to those of the broader international humanitarian system to ensure interoperability. USAID/OFDA's long-standing interagency agreements and partnerships are critical in mobilizing specialized and unique capabilities from across the U.S. Government onto the DART.

- **The Department of Health and Human Services (HHS)**: HHS Operating and Staff Divisions (including CDC, NIH, FDA, OASH/USPHS, OGA, and ASPR) can provide support in the following areas: technical and diplomatic engagement with, and in support of, the World Health Organization, engagement and information exchange with Ministries of Health and other government officials through existing bilateral relationships, the IHR (2005) National Focal Point and other critical bilateral and multilateral international partnerships, alignment of domestic public health emergency preparedness and response efforts, including research response, with the international response efforts (including the provision of

47

international assistance), participating or leading bilateral or multilateral epidemiologic and/or public health response efforts, making countermeasures available, including through research and development efforts, and mobilization/deployment HHS medical and public health assets, as necessary, including HHS MCM and HHS public health and medical personnel such as the Public Health Service Commissioned Corps or National Disaster Medical System, if needed. Specific operating and staff divisions contributions include:

o **The U.S. Centers for Disease Control and Prevention (CDC)**: Through its existing relationships CDC may facilitate requests for assistance from the host government. CDC will provide epidemiological expertise and technical assistance on disease outbreaks and control at the request of the host government. Because of CDC's role in the international community, CDC will likely be the first agency engaged and its technical leadership will need to be maintained to ensure the efficiency and efficacy of the U.S. Government response. In the capacity of outbreak response, in direct coordination with the respective Ministry of Health this could include but not be limited to activation of CDC's Emergency Operations Center, deployment of Global Rapid Response Teams, development or improvement in surveillance including laboratory capacity and distribution of diagnostics through the Laboratory Response Network and other networks, training in and performing of contact tracing, determination of risk factors, assistance in quarantine criteria, support in development of microplans for immunization activities.

o **The HHS Office of the Assistant Secretary for Preparedness and Response (HHS/ASPR)**: Provides leadership in international programs, initiatives, and policies that deal with public health and medical emergency preparedness and response.[6] HHS/ASPR manages the HHS Secretary's Operation Center and the U.S. International Health Regulations (IHR) (2005) National Focal Point (NFP). The NFP manages the U.S. assessment and notification process for domestic potential public health emergencies of international concern (PHEIC) as well as other emergency communications, including CBRN events, and the sharing of routine public health with the World Health Organization and other IHR NFPs worldwide. In addition, HHS/ASPR provides leadership for HHS activities during the U.S. CBRN response to an affected nation in close coordination with other U.S. Government agencies. HHS/ASPR's Biomedical Advanced Research and Development Authority (BARDA) can rapidly respond to accelerate development of medical and non-MCM, in collaboration with the National Institutes of Health (NIH) and DOD through the Public Health Emergency MCM Enterprise (PHEMCE). ASPR, in collaboration with the CDC and in coordination with the Secretary of Homeland Security, exercises the responsibilities and authorities of the HHS Secretary with respect to coordination of the Strategic National Stockpile (SNS), and along with CDC, NIH, FDA and OGA, advice on the international deployment of

---

[6] 42 U.S.C. 300hh-11(b)(6).

SNS assets.[7] ASPR has deployment authority for Federal (non-DOD) medical personnel (including the National Disaster Medical System (NDMS), and along with OGA and CDC, makes recommendations on the international deployment of HHS public health and medical personnel.[8] ASPR, along with CDC and stakeholders across HHS and the rest of the U.S. Government, also coordinates U.S. Government efforts to identify, obtain and coordinate distribution of samples of influenza and non-influenza pathogens with the potential to cause a public health emergency both domestically or internationally.[9] In response to an international event, ASPR capabilities that may support coordinating U.S. Government response efforts that include Mass Disaster Response (Direct Medical Care, Patient Evacuation Support, and Mass Fatality Management); Protect Responder/Worker Safety and Health; CBRN Public Health and Medical Consultation, Technical Assistance; and Health/Medical Equipment and Supplies (MCM including medical supplies, biologics, pharmaceuticals, blood products, vaccines and antitoxins).

- o **The National Institutes of Health (NIH)**: NIH will serve as the lead agency for the U.S. biomedical research response. NIH, through its 27 institutes and centers, supports and conducts a comprehensive biomedical research program including basic science, preclinical studies, and clinical trials to improve public health. NIH sponsored and conducted research on emerging and re-emerging infectious diseases extends from the bench to the bedside, and facilitates the discovery and development of MCM including diagnostics, therapeutics, and vaccines to prevent, treat, and control diseases in the U.S. and globally. NIH collaborates with host countries, academia, industry, and other U.S. Government agencies, as well as with international research institutions and organizations, to respond to international public health emergencies. Working collaboratively, NIH will lead development and implementation of the U.S. Government research agenda, including development of MCM, based on Ebola lessons learned (*HHS Ebola Improvement Plan*). Working with State and OGA, NIH will also represent the United States in the global research response, both in multilateral and bilateral forums and with partner countries. NIH will also ensure that research synergizes with other response actions, in collaboration with USAID/OFDA, CDC, and others. The research agenda will reflect the following priorities:

---

[7] *The Policy Framework for Responding to International Requests for Public Health Emergency Countermeasures from the U.S. Department of Health and Human Services* describes how the U.S. Government receives, considers, decides upon, and responds to international requests for the sharing of HHS public health emergency countermeasures, within existing legal and regulatory frameworks and current operational capabilities. As described in this document, there may be significant caveats to the ability of HHS to deploy these assets internationally under certain circumstances.

[8]HHS has developed internal policy documents which detail existing authorities and funding that HHS could use to deploy SNS assets and personnel. As described in these documents, there may be significant caveats to the ability of HHS to deploy these assets internationally under certain circumstances. *The Policy Framework for Responding to Requests for the International Deployment of Department of Health and Human Services Public Health and Medical Personnel* describes how HHS is to receive, analyze make decisions about, and respond to international requests for HHS public health and medical personnel during international medical and/or public health emergencies that warrant coordination among HHS offices and agencies and/or other U.S. Government departments and agencies.

[9] The DRAFT *United States Government Framework for the Rapid Sharing of Biological Material Related to Non-Influenza pathogens with the Potential to Cause a Public Health Emergency of International Concern* describes the process by which relevant Departments/Agencies within the U.S. Government jointly identify, obtain, and coordinate distribution of either domestic or international biological material related to non-influenza pathogens with the potential to cause a public health emergency.

identifying parameters of the health emergency, mitigating mortality and morbidity, ending the health emergency, and enhancing future emergency preparedness. NIH will work in close partnership with ASPR, ASPR/BARDA, FDA, CDC, DOD, and other agencies relevant in a particular emergency, such as USAID, USDA etc.

- **The Food and Drug Administration (FDA)**: FDA can provide assistance by working closely with manufacturers and U.S. government partners to expedite the development and availability of biologics (including vaccines), drugs, and devices (including diagnostic tests and personal protective equipment). FDA provides ongoing technical support to the World Health Organization and may provide support to regulatory authorities of affected countries to streamline development and expedite export and availability of countermeasures.

- **The Office of the Assistant Secretary for Health (OASH)**: OASH oversees 12 core public health offices — including the Office of the Surgeon General and the U.S. Public Health Service Commissioned Corps — a unique and deployable asset that is one of the seven uniformed services of the United States. Responsibilities include the ASH serving by statute as the Director of the National Vaccine Program and setting vaccination policy, and as the Director of the National Blood Safety Program. OASH helps coordinate the Department's response (both domestically and internationally) utilizing its key leadership including the Regional Health Offices, the Surgeon General, and the Commissioned Corps. OASH works with ASPR to make recommendations on international and domestic deployments. The international Ebola response, in particular, placed heavy emphasis on deployment of the Corps as the only U.S. government asset providing direct patient care to those potentially afflicted with Ebola Virus Disease.

  - **The HHS Office of Global Affairs (HHS/OGA)**: HHS/OGA serves as the primary point within HHS for setting priorities for international engagements and provides policy and diplomatic engagement, with, and in support of, WHO, engagement and information exchange with Ministries of Health and other government officials, and provide outreach on other critical bilateral and multilateral international partnerships.

- **The Department of Defense (DOD):** DOD can provide assistance and support response efforts, particularly relevant biosurveillance, biosecurity, mil-mil or mil-civ capacity building efforts, or relevant countermeasures research and development. Additional unique response capabilities can be provided if needed, such as logistics, transport, security, medical treatment when there are critical capacity gaps that cannot be easily filled by civilian actors. DOD also plays a key role in developing MCM, coordinated through the PHEMCE.

- **The U.S. Department of Agriculture (USDA):** USDA can support U.S. Government policy and diplomatic engagements with the World Organization for Animal Health (OIE) and/or the Food and Agriculture Organization (FAO) and, in coordination with Embassies, USDA can support engagements and information exchanges with Ministries of Agriculture and other government officials, especially to contribute to agricultural analyses and reporting on disease situations affecting the food and agriculture sector. Also, USDA has a mechanism to loan USDA experts to support the FAO Crisis Management Center – Animal Health's responses to animal disease emergencies in developing countries that request assistance. In addition, USDA, in concert with FDA, has an obligation to protect the domestic food supply, and would continue to monitor imports of food and food products to ensure their safety. USDA can also lead the U.S. research response to zoonotic diseases where the source of infection includes livestock and poultry. Working collaboratively with DOS, DOD, DHS, and NIH, USDA can lead the development and implementation of a U.S. Government agricultural research agenda, such as development of veterinary MCM and vector control to prevent and control the spread of vector-borne and zoonotic diseases in animal reservoirs. Working with international research institutions and global alliances, USDA can establish strategic research collaborations to help developing countries control and prevent diseases at the source. A research agenda could reflect priorities such as understanding the ecology of infectious diseases, preventing disease outbreaks, developing diagnostics and vaccines fit for purpose, and enhancing disease control programs.

- **The Department of Homeland Security (DHS):** DHS leads United States Government activities related to global health threats at U.S. borders and ports of entry, in conjunction with HHS, DOS, and USDA. Additionally, the National Biosurveillance Integration Center (NBIC), housed within the DHS Office of Health Affairs, provides shared situational awareness and enables early warning of emerging infectious diseases and acute biological events (both international and domestic) through collaboration with federal partners. NBIC provides regular biosurveillance updates and spot reports to federal, state, and local decision-makers.

- **The Department of Transportation (DOT):** Responsible for the safe and efficient movement of people and goods in transportation, including the operation of the National Air Space. Under the Hazardous Material Regulations ensures the safe movement of hazardous materials, including pathogens capable of causing disease, in transportation.

## ii. Domestic: See Appendix 6 of the Biological Incident Annex, also pasted below

| Organization | Resource Name | Description |
|---|---|---|
| USDA | Animal and Plant Health Inspection Service (APHIS) | Provides technical assistance and assists in coordinating with nonprofit and private organizations and government departments or agencies to support the rescue, care, shelter, and essential needs of owners and their household pets and service and assistance animals. Depending on the incident type, APHIS will coordinate with HHS, EPA, USACE, and/or FEMA to provide technical advice regarding disposal of animal carcasses. |
| USDA | Disaster Supplemental Nutrition Assistance Program (D-SNAP) | Through the D-SNAP, Food and Nutrition Services is able to quickly offer short-term food assistance benefits to families suffering in the wake of a disaster. Through D-SNAP, affected households use a simplified application. D-SNAP benefits are issued to eligible applicants within 72 hours, speeding assistance to disaster survivors and reducing the administrative burden on state agencies operating in post-disaster conditions. |
| USDA | National Animal Health Laboratory Network (NAHLN) | NAHLN laboratories perform routine diagnostic tests for endemic animal diseases as well as targeted surveillance and response testing for foreign animal diseases, protecting human health by decreasing the risk of zoonotic diseases (those that can affect animals and humans). |
| USDA | National Veterinary Stockpile | When a veterinary response is required, assets may be requested from the National Veterinary Stockpile, which is managed by USDA APHIS as a resource to address foreign animal disease in livestock and poultry. |
| DHS | BioWatch | BioWatch system consists of units that collect air samples in more than 30 cities and a network of local, state, and federal laboratories that analyze samples on a daily basis with a goal of providing warning of possible biological attacks within 12 to 36 hours of an agent's release. BioWatch has conducted 37 laboratory and 20 field audits to date. For more than 10 years, BioWatch has operated 24 hours a day, 365 days a year. |
| DHS | Domestic Communication Strategy | The Domestic Communication Strategy is a guidebook which provides options for public information strategies, complementing existing federal plans and strategic guidance documents, which may be employed in a domestic terrorist attack or a credible threat to the homeland. |
| DHS | Integrated Consortium of Laboratory Networks (ICLN) | ICLN provides for a federally coordinated and interoperable system of laboratory networks that provide timely, credible, and interpretable data in support of surveillance, early detection and effective consequence management for acts of terrorism and other major incidents requiring laboratory response capabilities. The ICLN is a partnership between nine federal agencies: Department of Defense (DOD), Department of Agriculture, Department of Energy, Department of Health and Human Services, Department of Homeland Security, Department of Interior, Department of Justice, Department of State, and Environmental Protection Agency. The ICLN includes the following networks: DOD Laboratory Network, Environmental Response Laboratory Network, Food Emergency Response Network, Laboratory Response Network, National Animal Health Laboratory Network, National Plant Diagnostic |

| Organization | Resource Name | Description |
|---|---|---|
| | | Network, and the Veterinary Laboratory Investigation and Response Network. |
| DHS | National Bioforensic Analysis Center (NBFAC) | Conducts bioforensic analysis of evidence from a biocrime or terrorist attack to attain a "biological fingerprint" to help investigators identify perpetrators and determine the origin and method of attack. NBFAC is designated by Presidential Directive to be the lead federal facility to conduct and facilitate the technical forensic analysis and interpretation of materials recovered following a biological attack in support of the appropriate lead federal agency. |
| DHS | National Biological Threat Characterization Center | Conducts studies and laboratory experiments to fill in information gaps to better understand current and future biological threats, to assess vulnerabilities and conduct risk assessments, and to determine potential impacts to guide the development of countermeasures such as detectors, drugs, vaccines, and decontamination technologies. |
| DHS | National Biosurveillance Integration System (NBIC) | The mission of NBIC is to enhance the capability of the Federal Government to— <br> • Rapidly identify, characterize, localize, and track a biological incident of national concern. <br> • Integrate and analyze data relating to human health, animal, plant, food, water, and environmental domains. <br> • Disseminate alerts and pertinent information. <br> • Oversee development and operation of the National Biosurveillance Integration System interagency community. |
| DHS | Surge Capacity Force | DHS Surge Capacity Force is organized into four tiers, for the purpose of prioritizing and providing for an informed selection of deployable human assets: <br> • Tier 1 – is comprised of FEMA Reservists with FEMA credentials. <br> • Tier 2 – is comprised of FEMA Permanent Full-Time Employees with FEMA credentials. <br> • Tier 3 – is comprised of DHS full-time federal employees. <br> • Tier 4 – is comprised of full-time or part-time federal employees from other federal departments and agencies. |
| DHS (CBP Laboratories and Scientific Services) | Weapons of Mass Destruction Response Teams | Provides level "A" hazardous material technical response capabilities. |
| DHS (NPPD) | Sector Specific Agency – HHS has area of responsibility for Healthcare and Public Health | The Sector Outreach and Programs Division builds stakeholder capacity and enhances critical infrastructure security and resilience through voluntary partnerships that provide key tools, resources, and partnerships. The division operates the council and stakeholder engagement mechanisms for the critical infrastructure security and resilience community. The division also serves as the sector-specific agency for 6 of the 16 critical infrastructure sectors and collaborates with the other 10. |
| DHS (NPPD/Federal Protective Service) | Hazardous Response Program | This program includes initial investigations of suspicious or threatening chemical, biological, radiological, nuclear, and explosive (CBRNE) incidents; conduction of CBRNE threat assessments; confirmations of unauthorized presence of CBRNE agents and materials; and the conduction of emergency operations. The Hazardous Response Program also provides evacuation support during CBRNE incidents, CBRNE mutual aid response through agreement and training assistance. The program is compliant with Occupational Safety and Health Administration and National Fire Protection Association guidance and regulations. |

| Organization | Resource Name | Description |
|---|---|---|
| DHS (FEMA) | Consequence Management Coordination Unit (CMCU) | In response to notification of a terrorist threat or actual incident, FEMA will activate the CMCU in support of FBI-led crisis management operations at the Weapons of Mass Destruction Strategic Group (WMDSG). Within the WMDSG, the FEMA staffs and manages the CMCU. This unit is also supported by federal technical capabilities provided through the DOE/NNSA, HHS, DOD, and DHS. As the principal advisory unit for consequence management considerations within the WMDSG, the CMCU provides recommended courses of action in light of ongoing and evolving operations. The CMCU provides a link between FBI-led crisis response and FEMA-coordinated consequence management response operations. |
| DHS (FEMA), DOJ (FBI), DOD, HHS, EPA | Domestic Emergency Support Team (DEST) | A rapidly deployable, interagency team responsible for providing expert advice and support to the FBI Special Agent in Charge concerning the Federal Government's capabilities in resolving a terrorist threat or incident. |
| DHS (FEMA) | National Ambulance Contract | The National Ambulance Contract is not to be used to transport contagious patients. |
| DHS (FEMA) | National – Incident Management Assistance Team (N-IMAT) | N-IMATs are trained on CBRN-related scenarios and will be FEMA's lead in the field to coordinate and integrate inter-jurisdictional response in support of the affected state(s) or U.S. territory(s). N-IMATs provide initial situational awareness for federal decision makers and support the initial establishment of a unified command. IMATs provide for multi-disciplinary needs of emergency management and may include members from the inter-agency community. |
| DHS (FEMA) | Interagency Modeling and Atmospheric Assessment Center (IMAAC) | The IMAAC provides a single point for the coordination and dissemination of federal atmospheric dispersion modeling and hazard prediction products that represent the federal position during actual or potential incidents involving hazardous material releases. Through plume modeling and analysis the IMAAC provides emergency responders and decision makers with predictions of hazards associated with atmospheric releases to aid in protecting the public and the environment. |
| DHS (USCG) | Marine Security Response Teams (MSRT) | MSRTs constitute the Coast Guard's Counter-Terrorism Advanced Interdiction force capable of executing higher risk law enforcement missions against opposed/hostile maritime threats including all CBRN threats. The MSRT is a quick response, ready assault force to conduct Short Notice Maritime Response operations. The MSRT is capable of interdicting, boarding, verifying CBRN and explosive threats, and when required, engaging in offensive operations against hostile threats. |
| DHS (USCG) | National Strike Force (NSF) | The NSF supports On Scene Coordinators, Lead Agency Incident Commanders, Operational Commanders, and Combatant Commanders with technical experts, specialized response equipment, and incident management skills to mitigate the effects of hazardous substance releases; oil discharges; and chemical, biological, radiological, and nuclear incidents. The NSF includes the National Strike Force Coordination Center; Atlantic, Gulf, and Pacific Strike Teams, Incident Management Assist Team, and Public Information Assist Team. |
| DOC (NOAA) | Air Resources Laboratory (ARL) | The ARL focuses its dispersion research on the development and improvement of sophisticated dispersion models and other tools for air quality and emergency response applications. This includes volcanic eruptions, forest fires, nuclear accidents, and homeland security incidents. ARL also designs and evaluates high resolution observing networks, develops instrumentation, and conducts tracer field studies to improve the accuracy of atmospheric transport and dispersion predictions. |

| Organization | Resource Name | Description |
|---|---|---|
| DOD | Military Aeromedical Evacuation (AE) | Patient movement by the DOD requires a request from a state or a federal department and the activation of the patient movement and definitive care components of the National Disaster Medical System (NDMS). Patient movement regulated by the Global Patient Movement Requirements Center (GPMRC) is conducted on fixed wing aircraft from an Aerial Port of Embarkation to an Aerial Port of Debarkation<br><br>The AE Patient Movement functions are coordinated by the Global Patient Movement Requirements Center (GPMRC), a unit of the U.S. Transportation Command, at Scott Air Force Base, Illinois. The GPMRC will collect casualty information from the states and determine patients' clearance for flight. DOD then matches the patients' needs with the aircraft, medical crew on board, and h a destination facility (also known as "patient regulation").<br><br>States may move patients using civilian or National Guard assets to hospitals within the state (presumably based on a state emergency plan) without the involvement of GPMRC. |
| DOD | CBRN Response Enterprise | The CBRN Response Enterprise is composed of both Active Component (Title 10) Federal, and Reserve Component (Title 10) (Reserve Component Title 10 could include federalized National Guard forces) elements with the mission of providing focused lifesaving capabilities with increased responsiveness for Defense Support of Civil Authorities. National Guard CBRN Response Enterprise elements include WMD Civil Support Teams, CBRN Enhanced Response Force Packages, and Homeland Response Forces. National Guard forces that have not been ordered into a Title 10 status are under state Governor, not Secretary of Defense, command and control. The Defense CBRN Response Force, and two Command and Control CBRN response elements are composed of active duty, National Guard, and Reserve forces allocated to USNORTHCOM to respond in a Title 10 status. |
| DOD | Defense Intelligence Agency/National Center for Medical Intelligence (NCMI) (HPAC) | The National Center for Medical Intelligence provides intelligence assessments of foreign health threats, including pandemic warning, to prevent strategic surprise across the broad threat spectrum. |
| DHS (USCG) | Marine Security Response Teams (MSRT) | MSRTs constitute the Coast Guard's Counter-Terrorism Advanced Interdiction force capable of executing higher risk law enforcement missions against opposed/hostile maritime threats including all CBRN threats. The MSRT is a quick response, ready assault force to conduct Short Notice Maritime Response operations. The MSRT is capable of interdicting, boarding, verifying CBRN and explosive threats, and when required, engaging in offensive operations against hostile threats. |
| DOI/USGS | USGS Environmental Health | The USGS Environmental Health Mission Area has the capability to develop models and tools for identifying, monitoring and assessing emerging environmental health threats and pathways for human and animal exposure. These activities build upon USGS's expertise in the hydrologic, atmospheric, geologic, and ecologic processes that affect the transport and fate of agents in the environment. |
| DOI/USGS | The USGS Western Fisheries Research Center (WFRC) | WFRC conducts research and diagnostics on high consequence disease of wild fish species, including diseases that can spill over into and result in economic impacts to US aquaculture. WFRC serves as an Office of International Enforcement Reference Laboratory that provides international expertise on infectious hematopoietic necrosis (a viral disease) and bacterial kidney disease of fish. |
| DOI/FWS | The FWS Wildlife Health Office | The FWS W Wildlife Health Office Conducts critical work in wildlife health and disease surveillance, response, and management. The Wildlife Health office comprises a network of wildlife health experts located across the country supporting refuges, wetland management districts, and other service programs by (a) providing technical advice |

| Organization | Resource Name | Description |
|---|---|---|
| | | about wildlife disease issues, (b) providing guidance on adapting management strategies to prevent wildlife diseases. (c) identifying health surveillance needs, (d) conducting research projects to determine best practices in disease prevention. (e) providing veterinary services for field activities, and (f) supporting emergency response efforts. |
| DOI/NPS | National Park Service (NPS) Wildlife Health Branch and Office of Public Health | The NPS Wildlife Health Branch provide professional veterinary consultation and technical assistance to aid parks in conserving wildlife, identifying and responding to zoonotic diseases in wildlife populations, and working closely with the NPS Office of Public Health and state and local health departments in zoonotic disease prevention and response. The NPS Office of Public Health is staffed by public health service officers including physicians, veterinarians, environmental health service officers and engineers that oversee food, drinking water, and wastewater safety in parks as well as assisting in zoonotic and vector-borne disease surveillance and responses in parks. |
| DOJ (FBI) | Hazardous Evidence Response Teams | These teams are FBI field teams trained, equipped, and authorized to collect CBRNE evidence in hazardous environments. |
| DOJ (FBI) | Weapons of Mass Destruction Strategic Group (WMDSG) | The WMDSG is an FBI-led interagency coordination mechanism to address the U.S. Government response to a terrorism incident involving radiological or nuclear threats to include the identification and deployment of specialized interagency elements used to support the Radiological Nuclear Search Operations in locating, identifying, and interdicting the threat. |
| EPA | CBRN Consequence Management Advisory Team | This team is the lead EPA special team for provision of scientific and technical support for all phases of environmental response to a CBRN incident, including health and safety, site characterization, environmental sampling and analysis, environmental monitoring, building, structure, and outdoor decontamination. waste treatment environmental cleanup, and clearance; manages the EPA's Airborne Spectral Photometric Environmental Collection Technology fixed-wing aircraft, which provides chemical/radiological data and deploys and operates mobile and fixed chemical and biological laboratories. |
| EPA. | Environmental Response Laboratory Network (ERLN) | ERLN provides capability to perform routine and emergency analysis of environmental samples. ERLN is integrated into the ICLN organization. |
| EPA | Environmental Response Team | This team Provides scientific and technical expertise for response to traditional chemicals and hazardous materials, including health and safety, environmental sampling, air monitoring, toxicology, risk assessment, waste treatment, contaminated water/scientific divers, and site decontamination and cleanup and provides field-analytical and real-time air monitoring for chemicals with the EPA mobile laboratories known as Trace Atmospheric Gas Analyzers. |
| EPA | National Criminal Enforcement Response Team | This team Provides technical, safety, hazardous evidence collection, and other forensic support to law enforcement in the instance of a WMD terrorist attack or environmental catastrophe. |
| EPA | National Response Team (NRT) | NRT is a national-level multi-agency coordination entity comprised of 15 federal agencies that provides technical assistance and resource and policy support to the federal On-Scene Coordinator during NCP and ESF #10 responses to oil and hazardous materials. |

| Organization | Resource Name | Description |
|---|---|---|
| EPA, DHS (USCG) | Regional Response Team (RRT) | RRTs are co-chaired by the EPA and USCG. A regional-level multi-agency coordination entity comprised of 15 federal agencies, state, and tribal representatives that provide technical assistance and resource support to the Federal On-Scene Coordinator during NCP and ESF #10 responses to oil and hazardous materials. |
| EPA, DHS (USCG) | On-Scene Coordinators (OSC) | OSCs coordinate the on-scene, tactical response to oil and hazardous substances incidents. Actions include assessment of the extent and nature of environmental contamination; assessment of environmental cleanup options; and implementation of environmental cleanup, including decontaminating buildings and structures and management of wastes. The EPA generally provides the federal OSC for incidents in inland areas, while the USCG provides the federal OSC for incidents in coastal areas. |
| HHS | Administration for Children and Families (ACF) | ACF promotes the self-sufficiency of individuals, families, and populations with access and functional needs prior to, during, and after disasters; Human Services Technical Assistance assets are utilized in the field to provide these services. |
| HHS | Aerial Ports of Embarkation | HHS National Disaster Medical System Teams provide critical care health care provider augmentation to federal transporters at aerial ports of embarkation to manage patients prior to flight. |
| HHS | Assistant Secretary for Preparedness and Response (ASPR) | ASPR leads the nation and its communities preparing for, responding to, and recovering from the adverse health effects of public health emergencies and disasters. ASPR focuses on preparedness, planning, response, and recovery; provides federal support, including medical professionals through ASPR's National Disaster Medical System, to augment state and local capabilities during an emergency or disaster; and leads the federal Health and Social Services RSF of the NDRF to assist locally led recovery efforts in the restoration of the public health, health care and social services networks of impacted communities. |
| HHS | Assistant Secretary for Public Affairs (ASPA) | The HHS ASPA assumes the lead in media response for public health, coordinated with and through the Joint Information Center. HHS ASPA coordinates the overall HHS Public Affairs planning, development, and implementation of emergency incident communications strategies and activities for the department. |
| HHS (ASPR) | At-Risk, Behavioral Health and Community Resilience | Provides subject matter expertise, education, and coordination to internal and external partners to ensure that the functional needs of at-risk individuals and behavioral health issues are integrated in the public health and medical emergency preparedness, response, and recovery activities of the nation to facilitate and promote community resilience and national health security. |
| HHS | Biomedical Advanced Research and Development Authority (BARDA) | BARDA, within the ASPR Office of HHS, provides an integrated, systematic approach to the development and purchase of the necessary vaccines, drugs, therapies, and diagnostic tools for public health medical emergencies. |
| HHS | Crisis Counseling Assistance and Training Program | This is a state grant program administered by HHS/Substance Abuse and Mental Health Services Administration and funded by the FEMA. |
| HHS | Disaster Medical Assistance Team (DMAT) | A DMAT is a group of professional and para-professional medical personnel (supported by a cadre of logistical and administrative staff) designed to provide medical care during a disaster or other incident. DMATs are designed to be a rapid-response element to supplement local medical care until other federal or contract resources can be mobilized, or the situation is resolved. |

| Organization | Resource Name | Description |
|---|---|---|
| HHS | Disaster Mortuary Operational Response Team (DMORT) | DMORTs are intermittent federal employees, each with a particular field of expertise, who are activated in the case of a disaster. The DMORTs are directed by ASPR/OEM/NDMS. Teams are composed of funeral directors, medical examiners, coroners, pathologists, forensic anthropologists, medical records technicians and transcribers, finger print specialists, forensic odonatologists, dental assistants, x-ray technicians, mental health specialists, computer professionals, administrative support staff, and security and investigative personnel. |
| HHS | Disaster Mortuary Operational Response Team-Weapons of Mass Destruction (DMORT-WMD) | The DMORT-WMD team is composed of intermittent federal employees from across the nation. The primary focus of DMORT-WMD is decontamination of bodies when death results from exposure to chemicals or radiation. DMORT-WMD is developing resources to respond to a mass disaster resulting from biological agents. However, this team might have difficulty in responding to such an incident if the deaths occur in multiple locations. |
| HHS | Disaster Portable Morgue Unit (DPMU) | DPMUs are staged at locations on the East and West coasts for immediate deployment in support of DMORT operations. The DPMU is a depository of equipment and supplies for deployment to a disaster site. It contains a complete morgue with designated workstations for each processing element and prepackaged equipment and supplies. |
| HHS | Emergency Management Group (EMG) | The EMG is a scalable team that is utilized every day at some operational level of intensity. Its organization is designed to be flexible and can expand as needed. The EMG is the established structure through which information and potential threats are received and decisions, including the deployment of an Incident Response Coordination Team, are made. The EMG operates within the principles of the Incident Command System and National Incident Management System. The EMG effectively operates 24/7 but can reach its full capacity with associated liaisons within four hours. |
| HHS | Federal Medical Station | Federal Medical Stations (FMSs) are modular and rapidly deployable, providing a platform for the care of displaced persons who have non-acute health-related needs that cannot be met in a shelter for the general population during an incident. |
| HHS | International Medical Surgical Response Team IMSuRT) | An IMSuRT comprises federal employees used on an intermittent basis to deploy to the site of a disaster or public health emergency and provide high quality, lifesaving surgical and critical care. IMSuRT-South is based in Miami-Fort Lauderdale-Palm Beach metropolitan area. IMSuRT-East is based in Boston, and IMSuRT-West is based in Seattle. |
| HHS | Incident Response Coordination Team (IRCT) | The IRCT and the IRCT-Forward act as the HHS agent's on-scene at emergency sites under the direction of the EMG. The IRCT directs and coordinates the activities of all HHS personnel deployed to the emergency site and assists state, local, tribal and other federal/government agencies as applicable. |
| HHS | Joint Patient Assessment and Tracking System Strike Team | This is a two-person strike team that will be deployed to aerial ports of embarkment, patient reception areas/casualty collection points, and destination locations to track patients through the system. |
| HHS | National Disaster Medical System (NDMS) | ASPR OEM NDMS provides deployable medical response teams to augment the nation's medical response capability and support SLTT authorities through three major missions: (1) provide emergency medical care support, (2) transport patients from the affected area to medical care locations remote from the affected areas, and (3) provide definitive medical care at NDMS civilian member hospitals. |

| Organization | Resource Name | Description |
|---|---|---|
| HHS | National Electronic Disease Surveillance System | This system facilitates electronically transferring public health surveillance data from the healthcare system to public health departments. It is a conduit for exchanging information that supports the National Notifiable Disaster Surveillance System. |
| HHS | National Institutes of Health (NIH) | NIH is made up of 27 different components called institutes and centers. Each has its own specific research agenda. All but three of these components receive their funding directly from Congress and administer their own budgets. |
| HHS | National Public Health Information Coalition | HHS will leverage a network of state and local health public health communicators to exchange information and increase the likelihood of consistent messaging and communication activities between federal and state or local governments regarding the emergency and its impact on health. |
| HHS | National Veterinary Response Team | This is a cadre of individuals within the NDMS who have professional expertise in areas of veterinary medicine, public health, and research. It is the primary federal resource for the treatment of injured or ill animals affected by disasters. |
| HHS | Regional Emergency Coordinators | ASPR's primary representatives throughout the country at the regional level; coordinates preparedness and response activities for public health and medical emergencies. |
| HHS | Secretary's Operations Center (SOC) | The SOC operates 24/7/365. The mission of the SOC is to serve as the focal point for synthesis of critical public health and medical information on behalf of the U.S. Government. |
| HHS (And Private Sector) | Certified Bio-Containment Units for Highly Infectious Diseases (Category A) | These include Emory University, Atlanta GA; Nebraska Medical Center, Omaha, NE; National Institutes of Health, Bethesda, MD; St. Patrick Hospital, Missoula, MT. |
| HHS (CDC) | CDC Emergency Operations Center (CDC-EOC) | The CDC EOC coordinates the deployment of CDC staff and the procurement and management of all equipment and supplies that CDC responders may need during their deployment. When activated for a response, the CDC EOC can accommodate up to 230 personnel per 8-hour shift to handle situations ranging from local interests to worldwide incidents. |
| HHS (CDC) | Epidemic Information Exchange (Epi-X) | CDC's secure, web-based communications network that serves as a powerful communications exchange between CDC, state and local health departments, poison control centers, and other public health professionals. The system provides rapid reporting, immediate notification, editorial support, and coordination of health investigations for public health professionals. |
| HHS (CDC) | Epidemic Intelligence Service (EIS) Officers | EIS officers work in many health departments in the United States or at the CDC through the CDC's Center of Surveillance, Epidemiology, and Laboratory Services and are dispatched to investigate possible epidemics, due to both natural and artificial causes, including *Bacillus anthracis* hantavirus West Nile virus, and the Ebola virus. |
| HHS (CDC) | Health Alert Network | CDC's primary method of sharing cleared information about urgent public health incidents with public information officers; federal, state, territorial, and local public health practitioners; clinicians; and public health laboratories. |
| HHS (CDC) | National Institute for Occupational Safety and Health (NIOSH) | NIOSH is the U.S. federal agency that conducts research and makes recommendations to prevent worker injury and illness. NIOSH can deploy a multidiscipline team to provide guidance and technical assistance on responder and worker safety and health. |

| Organization | Resource Name | Description |
|---|---|---|
| HHS (CDC) | Laboratory Response Network (LRN) | The LRN and its partners maintains an integrated national and international network of laboratories that are fully equipped to respond quickly to acts of chemical or biological threats, emerging infectious diseases, and other public health threats and emergencies. |
| HHS (CDC) | National Notifiable Disease Surveillance System (INNDSS) | NNDSS is a nationwide collaboration that enables all levels of public health—local, state, territorial, federal, and international—to share notifiable disease-related health information. Public health uses this information to monitor, control, and prevent the occurrence and spread of state-reportable and nationally notifiable infectious and noninfectious diseases and conditions. NNDSS is a multifaceted program that includes the surveillance system for collection, analysis, and sharing of health data. It also includes policies, laws, electronic messaging standards, people, partners, information systems, processes, and resources at the local, state, territorial, and national levels. |
| HHS (CDC) | Public Health Information Network | CDC's national initiative to increase the capacity of public health agencies to electronically exchange data and information across organizations and jurisdictions (e.g., clinical care to public health, public health to public health and public health to other federal agencies). To do so, the Network promotes the use of standards and defines functional and technical requirements for public health information exchange. |
| HHS (CDC/Agency for Toxic Substances and Disease Registry) | Rapid Response Registry Team | This survey instrument gives local and state entities a tool to register responders and other persons exposed to chemical, biological, or nuclear agents from a disaster. The survey instrument is a two-page form that can be distributed on paper or electronically. It can be implemented quickly to collect information rapidly to identify and locate victims and people displaced or affected by a disaster. |
| HHS (CDC) | Strategic National Stockpile (SNS) Push Packages | A SNS Push Packages is a cache of pharmaceuticals and medical supplies designed to provide rapid delivery of a broad array of assets for an undefined public health threat in the initial hours of an event. This cache is packed in cargo containers that can be delivered anywhere in the United States within 12 hours of the federal decision to deploy. |
| HHS (CDC) | Strategic National Stockpile: Managed Inventory (MI) | If the incident requires additional pharmaceuticals and/or medical supplies, follow-on MI supplies will be shipped to arrive within 24 to 36 hours. If the agent is well defined, VMI can be tailored to provide pharmaceuticals, supplies, and/or products specific to the suspected or confirmed agent(s). In this case, the VMI could act as the first option for immediate response from the SNS program. |
| HHS (FDA) | Regulated Products/Commodity Response Teams | Provides assistance to state and local health authorities or in the absence of state and local health investigators, assumes primary responsibility for evaluation and recovery of food service establishments and pharmacies |
| HHS (FDA) | Medical Countermeasures Initiative (MCMi) Office of Counterterrorism and Emerging Threats (OCET) | This office coordinates FDA's medical countermeasures development, availability, preparedness, and response." with "This office leads an FDA-wide initiative to coordinate medical countermeasure development, preparedness and response. FDA ensures that medical countermeasures (MCMs)—including drugs, vaccines and diagnostic tests—to counter CBRN and emerging disease threats are safe, effective, and secure. This includes coordinating research, setting deployment and use strategies, and facilitating access to MCMs |
| HHS (USPHS) | Applied Public Health Team (APHT) | APHT provides resources and assistance to local health authorities throughout the United States. Currently five APHTs, each of which is a work force comprising 47 USPHS-trained Commissioned Corps officer responders. Yet each APHT is scalable and capable of providing only those resources needed. Each APHT is also responsive; as a Tier 2 team the APHT can deploy within 36 hours of activation. |

| Organization | Resource Name | Description |
|---|---|---|
| HHS (USPHS) | Capital Area Provider | Providers who respond only in the National Capital Region – mass gatherings on the Mall; e.g., doctors, mid-levels, nurses. |
| HHS (USPHS) | Mental Health Team | The mental health team can respond nationwide; provides assessment, screening, and training for behavioral health issues; psychologists, psychiatrists, licensed clinical social workers. |
| HHS (USPHS) | National Incident Support Team (NIST) | The NIST consists of 72 USPHS-trained Commissioned Corps officer responders. Each NIST is scalable, and is capable of providing only those resources needed. NIST is a Tier 1 team and can deploy within 12 hours of activation. |
| HHS (USPHS) | Rapid Deployment Force (RDF) | There are currently five RDFs, each of which is a workforce comprising 105+ trained USPHS Commissioned Corps officer responders. Yet each RDF is scalable, and is capable of providing only those resources needed. The RDF is also responsive; as a Tier 1 team the RDF can deploy within 12 hours of activation. |
| HHS (USPHS) | Regional Incident Support Team (RIST) | RISTs provide rapid assessments and initial incident coordination resources and assistance to state, tribal, and local health authorities within defined regions of the United States. There are currently eleven RISTs, each of which is aligned with one of the HHS regions (including the National Capital Region). |
| HHS (USPHS) | Service Access Teams | Service Access Teams provide assistance to health care facilities and other entities where federally medically evacuated patients have been sent. |
| HHS (USPHS) | Tier 1 – USPHS-Commissioned Corps Response Groups | Tier 1 teams (RDFs, NISTs, and RISTs) have implicit concurrence on the part of their respective agencies for deployability within 12 hours. |
| HHS (USPHS) | Tier 2 – USPHS-Commissioned Corps Response Groups | Tier 2 officers are also formally rostered on response teams (APHTs, Mental Health Teams, Capital Area Provider Teams, and Services Access Teams) and maintain implicit agency concurrence for deployability within 36 hours. |
| HHS (USPHS) | Tier 3 – USPHS-Commissioned Corps Response Groups | Tier 3 officers are not rostered on specific teams and do not maintain implicit agency concurrence but are on call once within every five-month period—their activation requires agency concurrence at the time of deployment. |
| GSA | Public Building Services | GSA provides leasing specialists to find federal facility |
| United States Postal Inspection Service | United States Postal Inspection Service | Conducts biological surveillance for pathogens shipped through the mail. |
| Department of Veteran's Affairs (VA) | Federal Coordinating Centers | Federal Coordinating Centers are DOD or VA centers whose personnel recruit non-federal hospitals within approximately a 50-mile radius of the airport or military airfield where NDMS hospital inpatients from affected states will likely arrive and be triaged, received, and transported to NDMS partner hospitals for inpatient medical care |
| Department of Veteran's Affairs (VA) | Disaster Emergency Medical Personnel System | Veterans Health Administration's main deployment program for clinical and non-clinical staff to an emergency or disaster. This program may be used for an internal VA mission as well as supporting a mission after a Presidential Disaster Declaration under the NRF ESF #8 (Public Health and Medical Services). |

## III.   Sample Exercises

| Example 1:  Cholera Epidemic in Iraq | | | | | | |
|---|---|---|---|---|---|---|
| **Epidemiologic Rating**<br>Key Epidemiologic Indicators (#of cases, case detection rate, transmission potential, mode of transmission, severity of illness) | **1a.**<br>**Normal Ops** | **1b.**<br>**Elevated Threat**<br><br>Assessment:  Yellow<br><br>Growing number of cases, mortality rate within range, interventions available | **1c.**<br>**Credible Threat** | **2a.**<br>**Public Health Emergency / PHEIC** | **2b.**<br>**Worsening public health emergency indicators/ PHEIC** | **2c.**<br>**Improving public health emergency indicators/ PHEIC** |
| *Other Critical Dimensions* | | | | | | |
| Humanitarian/development impact Indicators (mortality, impact on health/econ system, vulnerable children, food security) | | Assessment:  Orange/ Heightened Concern<br><br>Cholera outbreak is symptom of worsening humanitarian situation due to conflict. Humanitarian actors are providing assistance and interventions available. Permanent solutions or water sanitation infrastructure not feasible due to conflict | | | | |
| Security/Political Stability Indicators (US relationship, conflict/ security, governance) | | Assessment:  Red/Crisis<br><br>Conflict situation, difficult to provide assistance | | | | |
| Transmission/outbreak/panic potential in the United States | | Assessment:  Green/Minimal concern<br><br>Very low transmission risk to the US and high capacity to prevent spread | | | | |
| **Overall Assessment:** | **Monitor:**  UN Agencies and humanitarian actors are accustomed to addressing cholera outbreaks, and the outbreak can be handled through HA channels.  Near term situation unlikely to change and provide opportunities for water and sanitation (wat/san) infrastructure. | | | | | |

| Example 2: Middle East Respiratory Syndrome-Coronavirus cases in Jordan | | | | | | |
|---|---|---|---|---|---|---|
| **Epidemiologic Rating** Key Epidemiologic Indicators (#of cases, case detection rate, transmission potential, mode of transmission, severity of illness) | **1a. Normal Ops** | **1b. Elevated Threat** Assessment: Yellow Sporadic reports of cases in hospital settings, transmission and mortality rates within range | **1c. Credible Threat** | **2a. Public Health Emergency / PHEIC** | **2b. Worsening public health emergency indicators/ PHEIC** | **2c. Improving public health emergency indicators/ PHEIC** |
| *Other Critical Dimensions* | | | | | | |
| Humanitarian/development impact Indicators (mortality, impact on health/econ system, vulnerable children, food security) | | Assessment: Green/Minimal Concern Cases are not causing widespread outbreaks or impacting development or overall health systems. Cases not detected in refugee camp areas or internally displaced persons camp areas | | | | |
| Security/Political Stability Indicators (US relationship, conflict/ security, governance) | | Assessment: Green/Minimal concern Overall stable government and system, strained due to neighboring conflicts | | | | |
| **Transmission/outbreak/panic potential in the United States** | | Assessment: Yellow/Elevated concern The US has diagnostic capacity and experience treating MERS case. Very low outbreak potential | | | | |
| **Overall Assessment**: | **Monitor:** The number of MERS-COV cases has been low and has not posed too high a burden on the Jordanian health system to date. Given the characteristics of MERS, the situation warrants monitoring but no other action needed. | | | | | |

| Example 3a: Ebola in West Africa in March, 2014 | | | | | | |
|---|---|---|---|---|---|---|
| **Epidemiologic** Rating<br>Key Epidemiologic Indicators (#of cases, case detection rate, transmission potential, mode of transmission, severity of illness) | **1a.**<br>**Normal Ops** | **1b.**<br>**Elevated Threat** | **1c.**<br>**Credible Threat**<br><br>Assessment: Yellow | **2a.**<br>**Public Health Emergency / PHEIC** | **2b.**<br>**Worsening public health emergency indicators/ PHEIC** | **2c.**<br>**Improving public health emergency indicators/ PHEIC** |
| *Other Critical Dimensions* | | | | | | |
| Humanitarian/development impact Indicators (mortality, impact on health/econ system, vulnerable children, food security) | | | Assessment: Yellow, elevated concern | | | |
| Security/Political Stability Indicators (US relationship, conflict/ security, governance) | | | Assessment: Green/Minimal concern<br><br>Overall stable | | | |
| Transmission/outbreak/panic potential in the United States | | | Assessment: Green/Minimal concern<br><br>The U.S. was not anticipating domestic cases | | | |
| **Overall Assessment:** | **Monitor:** Ebola outbreaks occurred occasionally in Africa in the past and were contained after an initial spread. WHO and CDC experts were already in the field. Expectation was that this outbreak would be contained quickly. | | | | | |

| Example 3b: Ebola in West Africa in August, 2014 | | | | | | |
|---|---|---|---|---|---|---|
| **Epidemiologic Rating** Key Epidemiologic Indicators (#of cases, case detection rate, transmission potential, mode of transmission, severity of illness) | **1a. Normal Ops** | **1b. Elevated Threat** | **1c. Credible Threat** | **2a. Public Health Emergency / PHEIC** | **2b. Worsening public health emergency indicators/ PHEIC** | **2c. Improving public health emergency indicators/ PHEIC** |
| *Other Critical Dimensions* | | | | | | |
| Humanitarian/development impact Indicators (mortality, impact on health/econ system, vulnerable children, food security) | | | | Assessment: Red | | |
| Security/Political Stability Indicators (US relationship, conflict/ security, governance) | | | | Assessment: Yellow | | |
| Transmission/outbreak/panic potential in the United States | | | | Assessment: Green | | |
| **Overall Assessment:** | **Monitor Public Health Response:** Growing concern that the outbreak was not contained and had spread to three countries. MSF's calls on the seriousness of the outbreak was growing. WHO had just finally declared a PHEIC which mobilized additional resources. The U.S. Government was contemplating options to accelerate the response including potential mobilization and structure of a USAID DART and option to deploy the US military. | | | | | |

65

| Example 3c: Ebola in West Africa in September, 2014 | | | | | | |
|---|---|---|---|---|---|---|
| Epidemiologic Rating<br><br>Key Epidemiologic Indicators (#of cases, case detection rate, transmission potential, mode of transmission, severity of illness) | 1a.<br>Normal Ops | 1b.<br>Elevated Threat | 1c.<br>Credible Threat | 2a.<br>Public Health Emergency / PHEIC | 2b.<br>Worsening public health emergency indicators/ PHEIC | 2c.<br>Improving public health emergency indicators/ PHEIC |
| *Other Critical Dimensions* | | | | | | |
| Humanitarian/development impact Indicators (mortality, impact on health/econ system, vulnerable children, food security) | | | | Assessment: Red | | |
| Security/Political Stability Indicators (US relationship, conflict/ security, governance) | | | | Assessment: Red | | |
| Transmission/outbreak/panic potential in the United States | | | | Assessment: Red | | |
| Overall Assessment: | Response: By September, it was clear that all humanitarian and public health response systems were completely overwhelmed and the outbreak was spreading and accelerating. Growing signals that regional security and stability were at risk, particularly following spread in Nigeria. Impact on flights, travel, and commerce were becoming apparent. Late September, panic was sparked in the United States following the Thomas Duncan case and subsequent spread to two nurses in Dallas, Texas. | | | | | |

66

## IV.   Communications

Internal and external communications are critical throughout the course of the response to an emerging pathogen.  Internal communication mechanisms are the Federal Government's operational communication resources and links for supporting response and recovery operations, which include pathways for coordinating support for public health and medical services. External communication mechanisms are public information and warning resources for public reception of and compliance with public health guidance, including guidance on personal protective measures and access to health and medical interventions.

Key Questions:

1.  How is information being shared across the Federal Government?
2.  How is information being shared with SLTT partners?
3.  What are the messages to convey to the public regarding risk, preparations, and availability of MCM?

### Internal Communication

HHS leads and coordinates all Federal communication, messaging, and release of public health and medical information both across the U.S. Government and internationally with the World Health Organization (WHO) and affected countries.  For internal U.S. Government communications, the HHS Secretary's Operation Center (SOC) is the primary national-level hub for situational awareness and information-sharing related to public health and medical response.

More broadly, DHS coordinates internal and external communications related to domestic incident management.  For internal U.S. Government communications, the DHS National Operations Center (NOC) is the primary national-level hub for domestic situational awareness, a common operating picture (COP), information fusion, and information sharing pertaining to domestic incident management.  To coordinate external communications related to an incident, DHS convenes the National Incident Communication Conference Line (NICCL) for Federal communicators to exchange critical and timely incident information and develop coordinated Federal messaging strategies related to an incident.

### External Communication

As the lead agency for health and medical information, HHS plays a primary role within the overarching framework provided by DHS in an emerging infectious disease response.  HHS coordinates communications information related to the public health and medical aspects of a response, particularly in a public health specific emergency.  The HHS Secretary is the primary spokesperson for the public health and medical response, supported by subject matter experts within HHS.

In the event of a terrorist incident, the FBI would be consulted before issuing sensitive media/press releases.

The White House Office of Communications provides strategic direction for public information and warning activities. During an early response requiring a coordinated Federal effort, the White House Office of Communications would provide strategic communications guidance and maintain overall authority over public information and warning activities.

## V.    Concept of Operations: Domestic Response

Responses to infectious disease outbreaks are primarily managed and monitored by public health agencies at the SLTT level of government. As incidents change in size, scope and complexity, a higher-level of coordination between public health, emergency management, and law enforcement communities may be required in the form of supplemental and complimentary support. The Public Health Agency at the local or state level should be deemed the lead response agency with HHS as the default LFA and originator for federal agency-to-agency operational support tasks during any biological incident. Many conceivable instances will not result in a Stafford Act declaration, yet, additional resources and coordination support may be facilitated by FEMA to deliver supplemental support to the lead public health agencies. Depending on the situation and in rare instances, other federal agencies may play a lead coordinating role with HHS retaining its lead functional responsibilities to deliver public health and medical capabilities.

Domestic public health and medical response and recovery occur in three phases: preparedness, response, and recovery.

| Phase 1 | | | Phase2 | | | Phase 3 |
|---|---|---|---|---|---|---|
| Primarily Pre-Incident | | | Begins when an Incident Occurs Upon Notification | | | Sustained Operations |
| 1a | 1b | 1c | 2a | 2b | 2c | 3a |
| Normal Operations | Increased Likelihood or Elevated Threat | Near Certainty or Credible Threat | Activation, Situational Assessment, and Movement | Employment of Resources and Stabilization | Intermediate Operations | Long-Term Recovery Operations |

In the event of a suspected or emerging biological incident (Phase 1c), the Federal Government may conduct enhanced public health surveillance and increase coordination among Federal partners and SLTT authorities. A Unified Coordination Group (UCG) may convene to facilitate information sharing and coordination. In this phase, DHS and HHS co-lead the UCG at the national level. If there is actionable intelligence of a deliberate incident, the FBI leads and coordinates law enforcement and investigative matters to counter the threat.

In conjunction with the national level, affected SLTT jurisdictions may engage with key stakeholders, including health departments, emergency management, law enforcement, environmental quality, and fusion centers in order to increase their information sharing and coordination. Early in a response, SLTT jurisdictions may also increase public health surveillance and sampling, develop public messaging strategies, and implement response plans. At the same time, affected SLTT jurisdictions maintain communications with Federal departments and agencies to provide situational awareness and to coordinate public messaging, as appropriate.

www.ingramcontent.com/pod-product-compliance
Lightning Source LLC
Chambersburg PA
CBHW041750190326

*9781608881864*